Quality Measurement

A Practical Guide for the Emergency Department

DERENDA S. PETE, RN, MBA

BUD PATE, REHS

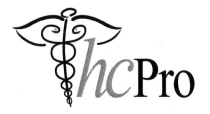

Quality Measurement: A Practical Guide for the Emergency Department is published by HCPro, Inc.

Derenda S. Pete, RN, MBA, Co-author
Bud Pate, REHS, Co-author
Ronald D. Moen, Reviewer
Peter Pronovost, MD, PhD, Reviewer
Amy Anthony, Managing Editor
Matthew Cann, Group Publisher
Mike Mirabello, Senior Graphic Artist
Paul Singer, Layout Artist
Jean St. Pierre, Creative Director
Tom Philbrook, Cover Designer
Suzanne Perney, Publisher

Advice given is general. Readers should consult professional counsel for specific legal, ethical, or clinical questions.

Arrangements can be made for quantity discounts. For more information, contact:

HCPro, Inc.
P.O. Box 1168
Marblehead, MA 01945
Telephone: 800/650-6787 or 781/639-1872
Fax: 781/639-2982
E-mail: *customerservice@hcpro.com*

Visit HCPro at its World Wide Web sites:
www.hcpro.com **and** *www.hcmarketplace.com*

Contents

Figures v

About the authors vii

About the reviewers ix

Introduction xi

Chapter one: How measurement contributes to new knowledge 1

The importance of common definitions 5
Benchmarking 6
Measurement principles 6
How measurement contributes to new knowledge 8
Current knowledge—the three questions 8
Cycle for learning and improvement—the PDSA cycle 9

Chapter two: Selecting and deselecting measures 11

Types of measures 14
Selecting measures 17
Deselecting measures 19
Case study—Selecting the correct indicators 20

Chapter three: Designing a new measure 25

What are you trying to measure? 27
How do you define the measure? 28
How good is the measure? 29
Case study—Choosing and developing boarder hours 30
Sample process measures for the ED 35

Chapter four: Creating a data collection and reporting system 37

Data collection. 39

Sampling 40

Other data collection issues 43

Displaying and analyzing the data 45

Ways to measure process times 57

Chapter five: Seven steps to uncorking the ED bottleneck by deploying effective scorecards 61

Focusing leadership's attention 63

The power of the scorecard. 64

Seven steps to scorecard nirvana 66

Chapter six: Understand the pros and cons of improvement methods . . . 79

The more things change the more they remain the same. 82

Definitions and distinctions 87

Case study—Lean Thinking: Finding the wheelchair 89

Influencing leadership's decision. 95

Appendix A: Evaluating measurement systems 97

Studying the quality of a measure. 100

Precision for classification data 101

Measurement discrimination and rounding of numbers. 104

More guidance on evaluating measurement systems 104

Appendix B: Additional case studies 105

Case study #1: First dose of antibiotics 107

Case study #2: Reconciliation of medications. 109

Appendix C: Glossary 111

Figures

Chapter one

Figure 1.1: Levels of systems 4
Figure 1.2: Model for improvement 9

Chapter two

Figure 2.1: Outcomes from a system 13
Figure 2.2: Output of a measurement process 15
Figure 2.3: Types of quantitative data 15
Figure 2.4: LWBS control chart 22
Figure 2.5: Patient flow scorecard 24

Chapter four

Figure 4.1: Average triage time based on ALL triages 41
Figure 4.2: Sample size run charts 42
Figure 4.3: Interfacility transfer data collection tool 44
Figure 4.4: Control chart for survey score 46
Figure 4.5: Spider diagram 47
Figure 4.6: Checklist for measures 48
Table 4.1: Steps to develop ED measures 49
Table 4.2: ED quality and performance measures 50
Table 4.3: Web sites for indicator selection and development 56
Figure 4.7: Distribution of times: Perfect distribution 58
Figure 4.8: Distribution of times: Typical distribution 58
Figure 4.9: From arrival to triage 59

Chapter five

Figure 5.1: Traditional scorecards for management accountability 64

Figure 5.2: Balanced scorecard—Clinical operations 65

Figure 5.3: Indicator matrix 68

Figure 5.4: Indicator worksheet 71

Figure 5.5: Sponsorship identification—Improvement of the triage process 74

Figure 5.6: Sponsorship identification—Improvement of nursing

report process to 3 North 75

Figure 5.7: Sponsorship identification—Improvement of physician

productivity in the ED 75

Figure 5.8: Sponsorship identification—Improvement of consultant response

time to the ED 76

Figure 5.9: Sponsorship identification—Improvement of radiology

turnaround time 76

Figure 5.10: Sample scorecard 78

Chapter six

Figure 6.1: Improvement cycles 83

Figure 6.2: Pareto analysis 84

Figure 6.3: Cause and effect or Ishikawa diagram 85

Figure 6.4: Sigma 88

Figure 6.5: Tracking the wheelchair hunt 91

Figure 6.6: Reducing non-value-added steps 92

Appendix A

Figure A.1: Measurement as a process 99

Figure A.2: Illustration of precision, bias, and accuracy with four

measurement process 102

Figure A.3: Measurement process evaluation 103

About the authors

Derenda S. Pete, RN, MBA

Derenda S. Pete, RN, MBA, is a nationally recognized healthcare facilitator and emergency services clinician with experience as a project director, senior consultant, healthcare administrator, and department manager. As a managing partner of InSight Advantage, she helps institutions across the country address difficult operational issues. By combining her knowledge of best demonstrated practices with profound data analysis skills and practical clinical/operational expertise, she guides her clients toward improved customer service and profitability. Her approach, which typically focuses on labor optimization and process redesign, has succeeded in maximizing her clients' functional capacity and improving their return on investment.

Derenda is also the co-creator of industry-leading departmental redesign software and review processes. She serves as faculty to Urgent Matters, an emergency department improvement effort organized by George Washington University and funded by a Robert Wood Johnson Foundation grant.

She was previously a paramedic and flight nurse associated with Herman Life Flight in Houston, Texas. She received her masters in business administration from Houston Baptist University and has worked with institutions across the country on behalf of such consulting firms as West Hudson, Empath, and Adams and Associates.

Bud Pate, REHS

Bud Pate, REHS, joined The Greeley Company after 15 years at Kaiser Permanente. Bud was responsible for a wide range of region-wide quality and compliance initiatives during his tenure at Kaiser in Southern California. He was responsible for standards and survey processes established by the Joint Commission on Accreditation of Healthcare Organizations (JCAHO), the Centers for Medicare & Medicaid Services, the California Department of Health Services, and the Office of Statewide Health Planning and Development.

Bud also held leadership roles in Kaiser teams that developed industry-leading processes for the integration of health plan and hospital credentialing, moderate and deep sedation, and best practice driven assessments of emergency departments.

Before joining Kaiser Permanente in 1988, Bud was the supervisor of the Acute and Ancillary Services Section of the Los Angeles County Department of Health Services, Health Facilities Division. In that role, he was responsible for state licensing and Medicare/Medicaid certification activities for more than 150 general acute care hospitals, 200 home health agencies, and several dialysis and surgery clinics. Bud taught epidemiology and Washington Technical Institute in Washington, DC, prior to joining the LA County DHS.

A nationally recognized expert in healthcare operations and compliance, Bud chaired the Joint Committee on Accreditation of the California Healthcare Association and regional healthcare councils for many years. Bud represented the American Hospital Association on JCAHO's Standards Review Task Force, the Hospital Advisory Committee, and other JCAHO work groups and panels that were part of the *Shared Visions—New Pathways*™ development effort.

Bud is a prolific and engaging speaker on a variety of topics, ranging from the JCAHO's survey process, mitigating emergency department overcrowding by improving patient flow, root cause analysis, the Emergency Medical Treatment and Active Labor Act, and other compliance and quality topics. He has lectured in many settings, including programs sponsored by the National Institute for Occupational Safety, the Institute for Healthcare Improvement, the University of California at Los Angeles, California State University in Northridge, and the California Medical Association. Bud has authored articles on accreditation and root cause analysis, including an article published by IHI on the diagnosis and treatment of blame. Bud's last effort (with Derenda Pete of InSight Advantage) is *Solving Emergency Department Overcrowding: Successful Approaches to a Chronic Problem,* a book that was published in 2003 by HCPro, Inc.

Bud received his Bachelor of Arts degree from the University of California at Los Angeles and a Certificate in Environmental Management from the University of Southern California, School of Public Administration. He is a Registered Environmental Health Specialist in the state of California.

About the reviewers

Peter J. Pronovost, MD, PhD

Peter J. Pronovost, MD, PhD, is an associate professor in the departments of anesthesiology/critical care medicine; surgery; and health policy/management at the Johns Hopkins University in Baltimore, MD. He is a practicing anesthesiologist and critical care specialist, with a PhD in clinical investigation from the graduate training program at the Johns Hopkins Bloomberg School of Public Health. His interest and expertise involves applying clinical research methods to improving quality of healthcare and safety, especially in intensive care units (ICU).

At Johns Hopkins, Dr. Pronovost is medical director of the Center for Innovations in Quality Care, director of inpatient care, co-chairs the Patient Safety Committee and directs performance improvement for intensive care units. Nationwide, he is chair of the ICU Advisory Panel for Quality Measures with JCAHO, chair of the ICU Physician Staffing Committee for the Leapfrog Group, is helping lead an effort to develop the ideal ICU design with the IHI, and developing standards for ICU quality.

Dr. Pronovost has written more than 100 articles in the fields of patient safety, ICU care, quality healthcare and evidence-based medicine.

Ronald D. Moen

Ronald D. Moen is a statistician, consultant, and teacher to industry, government, healthcare, and education. He is co-founder and partner of Associates in Process Improvement (API, 1984) and adjunct lecturer in the physics and engineering science department at the University of Michigan-Flint (since 1995). His experiences of over 30 years include General Motors Corporation and the U.S. Department of Agriculture. He served as a Deming helper at 70 of his four-day seminars (1983–1993). He has been working with the Institute for Healthcare Improvement since 1998 as an advisor in measurement for various collaboratives and redesign projects.

He has advanced degrees in mathematics and in statistics and has given over 60 presenta-
tions and technical papers throughout the United States, Canada, Mexico, Europe, and
Asia over the last 30 years. He received the Craig Award in 1988, 1990, and 1998 from
the Automotive Division of the American Society for Quality for outstanding technical
papers. He is co-author of the book Improving *Quality through Planned Experimentation,*
(McGraw-Hill, 1991) and the second edition, *Quality Improvement through Planned
Experimentation* (McGraw-Hill, 1998). He is the 2002 recipient of the Deming Medal.

Pronovost and Moen are the authors of the HCPro, Inc. book, *Quality Measurement: A
Practical Guide for the ICU,* 2003.

Introduction

Measurement is fundamental to improvement: It allows you to evaluate, make changes and reevaluate performance.

Therefore, the lack of a valid measurement is a barrier to learning. Too many improvement efforts don't define what they need to measure or lack a proper system to collect data—and either is like driving blind, without the benefit of any feedback to help you adjust your course. The goal of this book is to help you overcome this barrier by providing the tools you need to develop valid measures of your improvement efforts.

How to use this book

You may be familiar with the phrase "every system is perfectly designed to achieve exactly the results it gets." Measurement systems are no exception. The one you develop for collecting measures of quality will determine your success. This book will guide you in developing such a system with tools, examples, case studies, and tips to help you along the way.

This book also will help quality improvement teams develop a performance measurement system. For example, a group may want to improve medication safety but lack a way to measure it. The tools and techniques provided in this book will help the improvement team transform the concept of medication safety into a valid measure of quality.

Before proceeding, however, let's define some terms.

What is measurement?

Measurement is a process—made up of procedures, equipment, and personnel—whose output is recorded observation or data. A measurement system includes

- aim (purpose or use)

- attribute (characteristic or condition)
- item being measured (activity, event, person, process, product, or system)
- measure(s)
- method of collecting and analyzing the data

What is data?

Data are recorded observations, such as video or audio recordings or blood pressure readings. Data collectors must strive to obtain unbiased (i.e., free from error) measures. Part of the challenge is to develop a robust system that includes explicit definitions for the measure and data collection tools.

What is a quality measure in healthcare?

More than 30 years ago, Avedis Donabedian[1] proposed measuring the quality of healthcare by observing its structure, its processes, and its outcomes.

The Institute of Medicine (IOM) has defined healthcare quality as "the degree to which health services for individuals and populations increase the likelihood of desired health outcomes and are consistent with current professional knowledge." In a broad approach to measuring healthcare quality, the IOM's definition incorporates two of Donabedian's three elements:

1. Determining the effects of healthcare on desired outcomes, including a relative improvement in health, consumer evaluations, or experience of healthcare

2. Assessing the degree to which healthcare adheres to scientifically proven processes or those that professionals agree affect health or patient preference

The IOM also says that healthcare should be effective, safe, patient-centered, timely, efficient, and equitable. These aims should help those who want to enhance healthcare using broader dimensions to customize their improvements.

Quality measures help determine whether providers use proven techniques and avoid those that tend to cause harm. To make better quality-care decisions, varied audiences need quality measures for healthcare purchasing, utilization, regulatory accreditation and monitoring, and performance improvement. All of these quality measures should be important, scientifically sound, usable across settings, and feasible.

Such measures provide insights into many aspects of quality. Peter Pronovost, one of this book's reviewers, offers the following example: "My six-year-old son Ethan had to make a collage about himself. We pasted pictures of Ethan with his sister and parents at the beach, at camp, and at school. Some of the pictures were clear. Others were granular. Some were important to Ethan. Others were important to his parents, his grandparents, and teachers. While no single picture allowed us to know Ethan very well, by viewing all the pictures together, we began to know him."

Like the pictures in Ethan's collage, quality measures help you see from various angles the level of care provided. Through this combined view, you see the full combined impact of the many facets of quality. As such, it may be more appropriate to refer to the "qualities" of care.

What is quality improvement?

A measurement system must fit into a process for quality improvement. There are three key components of an improvement system:

1. Caregivers must wish to work cooperatively for improvement.

2. There must be ideas or hypotheses about changes to the current system of care.

3. There must be a model for testing changes and carrying out those that result in improvement. Therefore, the ability to measure and to know if a change makes a process better is fundamental to any improvement system.

The importance of measuring quality properly

The goals of measurement are to develop new knowledge and to increase the rate of learning, and you accomplish these goals by measuring, implementing interventions, and re-measuring. However, even though it sounds simple, these steps are not taken often enough.

Most improvement efforts that fail do so for two reasons:

1. The improvement effort lacks an empowered team of knowledgeable front-line staff or senior leaders willing to allocate the necessary resources.

2. The team may not measure quality properly.

This book provides a guide to help you avoid the second reason.

You need valid measurement to tell you how you're doing in your efforts. For example, if you want to mark your child's height on a growth chart, you need a valid tool such as a ruler to measure height. You also need a valid way to measure—your child needs to take off his or her shoes and stand up straight. If the child stands on his or her tiptoes, he or she may introduce error.

The need for a valid outcome measure is the same in research and performance improvement efforts. Both address similar issues, and both need a valid measure of performance. They differ only in how they control against error and how they analyze data.

One kind of error, often called "systematic error," occurs when differences in patient characteristics rather than deviations in response to the intervention impact the study results. For example, assume that older patients are more likely to receive an intervention and, because of their advanced age, are also more likely to have a higher death rate. During a clinical study, if the intervention group has more elderly patients than the control group, you may incorrectly ascribe an increased mortality rate in the intervention group to the treatment rather than to the age of the patients.

In clinical research, assume that the greatest source of error is variation among patients. Control for these differences by matching, stratifying, randomizing, analyzing, and using regression techniques.

You also introduce error when you extrapolate your results into the future. Extrapolation occurs when you apply the interventions into varying conditions that occur over time. Quality improvement efforts are more concerned with time as a source of bias. And so evaluate small samples of patients over time and test them under varied conditions. Unfortunately, clinical research often ignores the error introduced by extrapolating results into the future or when applying the interventions to conditions.

It's also important to measure quality properly because consumers, purchasers, regulators, accreditation professionals, and insurers all require that caregivers measure performance accurately. Most importantly, however, is that your patients and communities need the best care possible. You must continuously learn and improve, and measurement will guide you in the right direction.

Reference

1. Avedis Donabedian, *Aspects of Medical Care Administration: Specifying Requirements for Health Care* (1973), (Cambridge, MA: Harvard University Press, 1973).

CHAPTER ONE

How measurement contributes to new knowledge

How measurement contributes to new knowledge

Length and weight measurements were made in Egypt as early as 3000 BC. The measurement of "how many" began when the Egyptians, Greeks, and Romans developed numeral systems. Around 600 AD, Hindus developed the decimal numeration system by adding the concept of place value and a symbol that meant "not any."

The concept of measurement slowly made its way to healthcare. For centuries, England gathered data on the death rates of hospital patients. Florence Nightingale (1820–1910) pioneered quality improvement by using data as a basis for action in order to reduce death rates. Boston surgeon Ernest Codman, MD, (1869–1941) was an early American proponent of monitoring and improving outcomes of surgical care.

Continued changes over the past 20 years have brought quality, measurement, and a philosophy of continual improvement to healthcare. However, the lack of valid measures to accelerate individual and team learning has been a great barrier to recent improvement efforts.

This book will guide you in developing measures to enhance learning and to result in better patient outcomes. In this book, we apply measurement to groups of patients, rather than to individual patients—the latter involves clinical decision-making that is beyond our scope here. Nevertheless, many of the principles for measuring groups also apply to individual patients.

This book focuses on interpreting collective data and determining the level of group you will measure, which you'll determine based on what will optimize learning. For example, you can combine data to include the level of individual physicians, the emergency department (ED), multiple hospitals within a system, and an entire health system (i.e., a country). But first you must collect data at the smallest unit level or it will be difficult to separate the data later.

For example, if a hospital system has four EDs and you only collect data at the hospital level, you cannot evaluate interventions within a specific ED. The data collection should therefore include information on whatever unit you want to evaluate. Figure 1.1 illustrates the levels of systems to which this book applies.

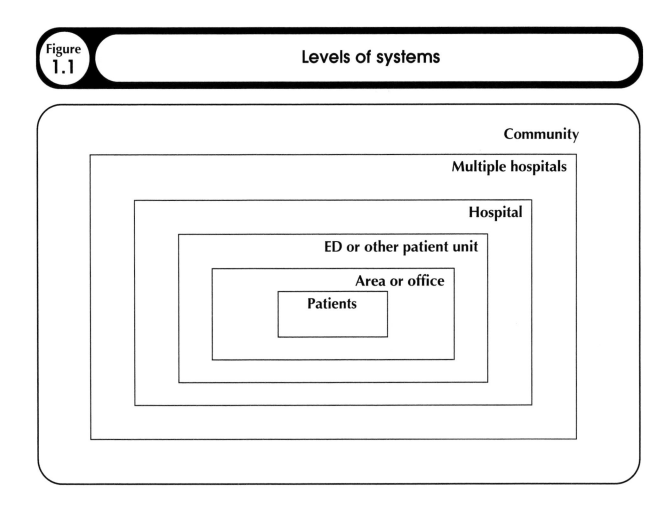

Figure 1.1 — Levels of systems

Community

Multiple hospitals

Hospital

ED or other patient unit

Area or office

Patients

Why do caregivers and researchers need to develop their own measures of quality, especially when the National Quality Forum and the Joint Commission on Accreditation of Healthcare Organizations are developing national measures? The answer is that you need more measures than those developed by these organizations.

You are faced daily with questions of what works and what does not. Therefore, as caregivers, you need to develop measures in your local work environment, carry out interventions, and evaluate their impact. Without these tools, you will inhibit your ability to learn and improve.

There are many areas you can measure. Examples include the following:

- How does a change in visiting hours improve family satisfaction?
- Did a training program improve pain management?
- Did the new fax machine improve the time for medication delivery?

There are hundreds of opportunities to conduct daily measures. Our goal is to help you determine what to measure and how to measure it.

The importance of common definitions

For a measure to be useful, it must have standard definitions.

The medical record is a measurement system, but you generally learn little from it because it has standardized measures for certain data points but not for others. First, to find an average weight of a patient, you need a standard definition of weight. You must then decide whether to use admission weight, idealized weight, current weight, or dry weight. You also need a standard method for obtaining weight. Should you use the weight from the history? If so, will it be based on the patient or on a relative's history? Or should you rely instead on the weight from the medical record, a bedside scale, a scale built into the bed, or a formula based on height and abdominal circumference?

You can use any of these methods. It is far more important—and is, in fact, necessary—to standardize a definition and a method to measure weight than it is to argue over which measure is more accurate. Aggregate data of an average weight is only meaningful if you use standard definitions and data-collection tools.

Benchmarking

Having common definitions and methods of measurement is increasingly important when you compare your results with those of other organizations. Benchmarking is the process of comparing ideas, interventions, and outcomes with others. It helps generate new ideas and concepts that may be adapted for use in the improvement efforts of an organization.

Even with common definitions and methods, however, the value of benchmarking may be limited to one hospital over time. In our experience, benchmarking in healthcare is used more to judge than to learn. There are a few examples of one healthcare organization identifying another that performed exceedingly well, replicating its process exactly, and improving performance. That is because, although concepts can be copied, interventions need local modification.

The limited value of benchmarking isn't surprising. Organizations differ in the skill of their individual caregivers, use of protocols, teamwork climate, leadership support, and information infrastructure. Each of these could affect whether an intervention identified in one organization could be used to improve the performance of another.

Measurement principles

There are five principles that will help you with measurement. They are as follows:

1. There is no true value of any characteristic that is defined in terms of measurement. Change the method of measurement and you change the result.
   —*W. Edwards Deming*

The point here is that measurement is relative. For example, you can determine a child's height using a tape measure on the wall, a 12-inch ruler, or a scale like the one used in a doctor's office. Each one, however, will produce a slightly different measure. Which is correct? All are. What is important is that you select a common method of measurement and use it consistently.

2. Our theories determine what we measure.
   —*Albert Einstein*

The decision on what to measure doesn't take place in a vacuum. Your experiences influence how you view the world, because you perceive it based on theories or conceptual models you know.

3. Scales and units of measures are chosen to optimize the learning of the user.
   —*Walter Shewhart*

This is a fundamental issue in measurement for improvement. You often have many options available. For example, should the unit of analysis be one day, one week, one month, or one year? The decision is determined by what optimizes learning. That is, the unit should be small enough that you can both provide frequent feedback and evaluate the effect of interventions.

4. There is no need for measurement if the intended use is strictly historical.
   —*W. Edwards Deming*

You measure to learn so that you can improve performance. But there is no point to measurement if your goal is solely to evaluate past performance and not apply what you learn to developing new interventions. View the process as a means to improve, not as an end in itself.

5. Statistical control (stability) of the process of measurement is vital; otherwise, there is no meaningful measurement.
   —*W. Edwards Deming*

With measurement, try to determine whether an activity leads to an improvement (either in a process or in the outcome). If there is wide difference in baseline performance, however, variation among patients will be greater than the improvement introduced by the intervention, which makes it very difficult to detect improvement.

Take an analogy from signal engineering. Let's say you want to determine whether a signal beacon is beeping. If you go into a soundproof room, it is easy to hear. But if you go into a wind tunnel, the background noise will limit your ability to hear the beep. Therefore, without a stable measurement process, you can't evaluate the impact of an intervention.

How measurement contributes to new knowledge

Creating the proper environment for learning starts with getting buy-in from executives, the team, and the staff. It also requires that the team have a clear direction, adequate human and capital resources, the right skills, and a supportive reward system. Most important, teams need a common road map—a model for learning and improvement that integrates measurement to acquire knowledge.

One of the more successful models for improvement in healthcare is given in Figure 1.2. The model has two components: current knowledge and the plan-do-study-act (PDSA) cycle for learning and improvement. This model represents a framework for improvement that is widely applicable and easy to use.[1] It helps you decide which actions to take and which not to take— based on existing knowledge—to meet the chosen objectives. As you take action and study the effects, the body of useful knowledge grows and enhances the power of those actions.

Current knowledge—the three questions

The following three questions form the first component of the model:

1. What are we trying to accomplish?
2. How will we know that a change is an improvement?
3. What changes can we make that will result in improvement?

The answer to the first question provides a goal for the improvement effort to keep it focused. To answer the second question, you must identify measures. This provides the foundation for learning that is fundamental to improvement. Answering the third question requires some ideas for change, such as an intervention or idea for improvement. The knowledge to support an idea may already exist, or it may help develop an idea for change. These three questions define the endpoint. Therefore, any effort to improve something would result in answers to these questions.

Figure 1.2

Model for improvement

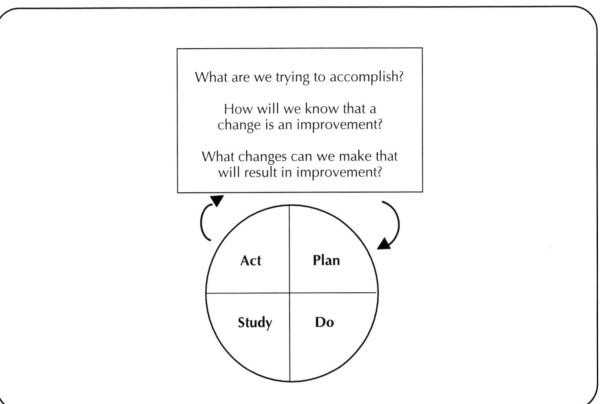

What are we trying to accomplish?

How will we know that a change is an improvement?

What changes can we make that will result in improvement?

Act   Plan

Study   Do

Cycle for learning and improvement—the PDSA cycle

The second component of the model is the PDSA cycle, which is an adaptation of the scientific method. Using it will enhance learning about the product, process, or system.

The PDSA cycle is used primarily to test and implement changes. Will the change result in improved performance of the product, process, or system in the future? What additional knowledge is necessary to take action?

The PDSA cycle is a vehicle for learning. A deduction (prediction) based on some theory is made, and then observation is taken (data collection). Next, the data is compared to the predicted consequences. A modification of the theory (learning) is done when the consequences and the data fail to agree.

Knowledge becomes useful when it results in action. People often have preconceived notions of the course of action and search for data to support it. The obvious danger here is that no learning takes place; hence, improvements in quality may not result.

Successful improvement and research teams navigate well through the road map described earlier. These teams desire new knowledge and have the support from leaders and front-line staff and resources, such as a project manager, research assistant, or analyst.

The next chapter provides detail on selecting measures that will help answer the second question in the model: "How will we know that a change is an improvement?"

Reference

1. G. J. Langley, K. M.Nolan, T. W. Nolan, C. L. Norman, and L. P. Provost, *The Improvement Guide,* (San Francisco: Jossey-Bass, 1996).

CHAPTER TWO

Selecting and deselecting measures

Selecting and deselecting measures

Measures should provide feedback that indicates whether changes to the healthcare system have resulted in improvements. Figure 2.1 illustrates examples of outcomes from various levels of systems.

Figure 2.1 — Outcomes from a system

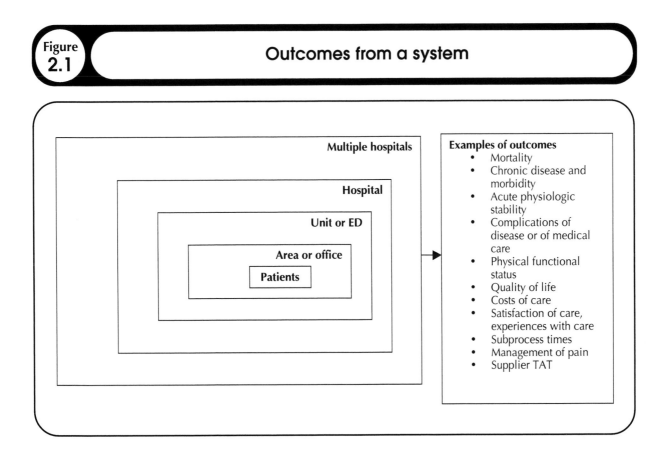

You can determine a measure of outcome, such as admission, by interpreting the appropriate aggregate data for the various levels of the system. For each outcome measure, there may be one or more surrogates, otherwise known as upstream process measures. These are often diagnostic and provide faster feedback and greater opportunities for learning.

The model for improvement (defined and illustrated in Figure 1.2 in **Chapter one**) can help you develop, test, and effect changes. These changes can occur at various levels of systems and improve one or more process measures or outcome measures. Define these measures by answering question No. 2 in the model for improvement, "How will we know that a change is an improvement?"

The outcome is always subject to two kinds of variation:

1. Variation in the process or system
2. Variation contributed by the measurement process

This second source of variation is always present (measurement principle No. 1 in **Chapter one:** There is no true value of any characteristic that is defined in terms of measurement. Change the method of measurement and you change the result. Consider this analogy: You look through a window to see the outside world. Selecting the best measure is analogous to finding the window that allows you the clearest view. Your goal is to find the best window—but you are always looking through a window.

Types of measures

Measurement is a process that produces outputs of data (recorded observations), with each measure resulting in a different output. The data may be quantitative (using numbers) or qualitative (without numbers, such as pictures, video, recorded sound, text, etc.). Qualitative data may be subjective determinations made by people using one or more of the senses (sight, sound, touch, smell, taste). See Figure 2.2 for an illustration of the measurement process with output.

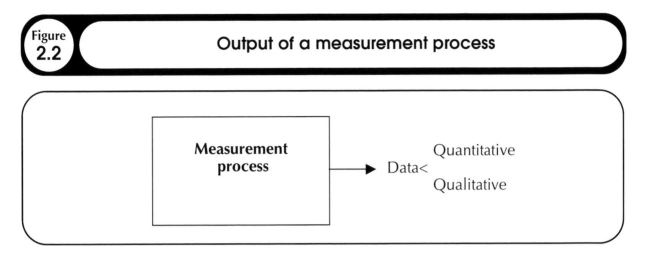

Figure 2.2 — Output of a measurement process

You can group quantitative data into different types, depending on the scale. Figure 2.3 shows examples of each.

Figure 2.3 — Types of quantitative data

Data type:	Nominal	Ordinal	Count	Ratio	Interval
Examples:	Medical diagnosis: gastroenteritis, N/V/D	Critical, serious, stable	# ED patients	% of patients with ab pain % of patients with hydration therapy	Patient weight, average length of stay

Note 1: In ratio data, zero means absence of the property of interest.

Note 2: Count, ratio, and interval data can usually be converted to ordinal or nominal data, but not the other way around.

Nominal data includes strictly categories or classes of some characteristic of interest, such as color or diagnosis. There is no order in nominal data. Ordinal data, however, provides a relative magnitude (e.g., more ill or less ill). Interval data is based on a continuous numeric scale (on it, zero has no specific meaning—it's just a value in the scale of numbers, like 6.3).

There are two types of ratio data. The first is a proportion: the number of events of interest (numerator) divided by the total population of interest (denominator). For example, the ED admission rate is a proportion often defined as the number of admissions divided by the total number of ED visits. The second type of ratio scale is a rate: the number of events over a specified time (numerator) divided by the population at risk for that event over time (denominator). For example, admissions per year per 1000 health plan members.

For either type of ratio, you need explicit definitions for both numerators and denominators. In addition, the numerator must come from the denominator.

An advantage of determining the rate is that rates incorporate exposure time, which enables you to make risk adjustment. For example, one of your measures may be thrombolytics therapy adverse reactions. What should the denominator be? You could make it a patient and, thus, a proportion (the number of patients with adverse reactions post-thrombolytics divided by the total number of patients). Nevertheless, only patients with thrombolytics risk having adverse reactions. Therefore, you would expect that since EDs have more thrombolytics events, they will have a higher proportion of patients with adverse reactions than those units with fewer thrombolytic events.

You can overcome this potential bias by changing your measure to a rate. Make the denominator the number of thrombolytics events, rather than a patient. Because a thrombolytic event is the exposure risk, using this measure accounts for variation in risk among EDs.

These same principles apply when measuring timely delivery (within 30 minutes of order written) of antibiotics. The risk of complications varies with the time a patient does not receive timely antibiotic therapy. So an appropriate numerator is the number of antibiotic delivered within 30 minutes of order written and the denominator would be the volume of antibiotic orders rather than patients. The popular Six Sigma improvement method expresses ratios in terms of "opportunities"—a patient may have many opportunities for adverse reactions, infections, etc.

Selecting measures

The simplest way to improve your measurement system is to use existing measures. To select the appropriate ones, ask the following:

1. What are you trying to measure?

This question asks you to define the concept to be measured, what is to be measured (e.g., experimental unit, specimen, patient, or organ), and how the measure will be used.

People use measures to

- learn and improve
- judge or make decisions
- monitor a change in condition

The need for risk adjustment increases when using the measurement for external regulators or public benchmarking, (e.g., ORYX core measures).

What concepts should an organization measure if the aim is improvement? Consider the following six dimensions of healthcare, as defined by the Institute of Medicine (IOM)[1]:

1. **Safety:** Avoid injuries to patients from care meant to help them

2. **Effectiveness:** Provide services to all who could benefit based on scientific knowledge and refrain from providing services to those unlikely to benefit (avoid underuse and overuse, respectively)

3. **Patient-centered:** Provide care that meets patient preferences, needs, and values, and ensures that patient values guide all clinical decisions

4. **Timely:** Reduce waits and delays for those who receive and give care

5. **Efficiency:** Avoid waste of equipment, supplies, ideas, and energy

6. **Equity:** Provide care that does not vary in quality because of sex, ethnicity, geography, and socio-economic status

Always take these six considerations into account when answering question No. 1, What are you trying to measure? As a whole, they are complementary and synergistic. There may be occasional conflicts among them, however, and it may be necessary to balance opposing objectives. You may also need different measures to evaluate each dimension.

2. How do you define the measure?

Standardize the measure by defining the concepts in operational procedures or specifications that everyone can understand. Consider the following when selecting a measure:

- What data type will allow you to attach a value to the concept?
- What is the plan for collecting the data? How often? How much?
- What is the level of aggregation?

Like a reporter, answer the who, what, where, when, and how of a measure.

3. How good is the measure?

Consider the quality of the measure. The first step is to test whether the measure has face validity for the user. That is, will the people using the data believe it's a good measure?

Another concern is the stability of the measurement, meaning that any variation is predictable within bounds. Without stability, a measurement is meaningless (see measurement principle No. 5 in **Chapter one)**. This variation, known as common cause variation, includes causes that are inherent in the process over time and is absent of any special causes. Establish the stability of the measure before evaluating other quality characteristics. To do so, display your data in a control chart, which will be discussed in **Chapter four.**

Also improve existing measurement systems for precision, bias, and accuracy. They are defined as follows:

- **Accuracy** is the degree of variation in individual measurements from the accepted standard value

- **Bias** is the amount of deviation of the average individual measurements from the accepted standard value

- **Precision** is the degree of variation in individual measurements from the same entity being measured

You can minimize the effect of variation by using good calibration practices to control bias (systematic error) and by repeating measures to increase precision (repeatability).

The user should define what "good" means, depending on how he or she will use the measure. For example, "good" could mean simple, inexpensive, accurate, precise, stable, reliable, or sensitive. When using a measure for benchmarking, the definition must be precise and valid.

Deselecting measures

The easiest decision for deselecting a measure comes from measurement principle No. 4 from **Chapter one**—There is no need for measurement if the intended use is strictly historical. Experience has shown that many measurements don't result in action. A simple test is to discontinue the measurement for a month and see whether anyone complains.

Another reason for deselecting a measure is because it is highly correlated with another one. A simple scatter diagram that plots two variables on an x/y graph of the two measures should reveal any correlation.

Some measures don't answer the third question of "How good is the measure?" Replace any measures that don't answer the question. Also, before you to select any measure, consider its contribution to a larger set of measures. Ask whether it provides balance to the set. See **Chapter four** for more about a balanced set of measures and deselecting non-value-added measures.

Case study

Selecting the correct indicators

Indicators for improvement v. trigger or screening indicators

We worked with a number of EDs to identify indicators that support ongoing improvements and other indicators that trigger more intensive reviews.

Left without being seen (LWBS) as a proxy for wait times and satisfaction

It's best to measure satisfaction and wait times directly. It's next best to use LWBS data wisely.

All EDs are (or should be) concerned about prolonged waits for care, which adversely affect quality and patient satisfaction. EDs usually are not able to easily or consistently collect wait times, but just about every hospital measures the number of patients who LWBS—it's part of their ED logging process.

Some departments call this disposition code "left prior to examination" or "left prior to the conclusion of care." Other departments subdivide this population into patients who leave at various points during the stay, such as "left prior to bed placement," "eloped," or "left against medical advice."

One advantage to using LWBS as a process measure is that no sampling is required. The department knows with certainty how many patients visited yesterday, how many were admitted, how many were discharged, and how many left before their care process could be completed. These numbers are low-hanging fruit indeed and therefore should be harvested.

Using LWBS data

Many hospitals with front-end problems trend the number of patients who LWBS as a daily percentage of visits; it has proven to be a very effective approach. We'll use one client hospital as an example.

Case study (cont.)

LWBS data sheds light on EMTALA compliance

This hospital had significant difficulties solving its EMTALA[2] woes. Medicare representatives repeatedly cited the hospital for failing to see patients as quickly as indicated by their complaint or triage category. The logic behind the citations, which was sustained by Centers for Medicaid & Medicare Services (CMS), was that medical screening delayed is medical screening denied.

At first the hospital used a compliance expert to review a sampling of charts to discover potential EMTALA problems. But no matter how many anecdotes about potential compliance problems were collected and studied, the underlying clinical intake processes did not improve.

The department did not have direct process times such as "time from presentation to provider for 'urgent' patients" (see case study in **Chapter four**), but like all EDs, it collected data on the number of patients who LWBS. One day it occurred to someone to take the number of LWBS patients and plot them on a control chart as a daily percentage, and the results were like magic:

> ✓ Staff members could see the impact of their changes
> ✓ LWBS percentage served as a proxy for wait times and satisfaction
> ✓ Leadership began to correlate daily LWBS rates with sick calls

And the department began to turn around.

A note of caution, however, trending LWBS data can be informative and useful, but it has limitations. There will always be an underlying percentage of patients who choose to leave rather than stay, no matter how short the wait time or how wonderful the service; they get scared, they feel better, they call their private doctor who makes an appointment, etc.

It is best to have a reliable triage system and to measure the wait times for "urgent" or mid-level patients (more about this indicator later).

Case study (cont.)

How to collect, analyze, and report LWBS rates

This medical center turned spotty LWBS rates into a meaningful driver for improvements.

1. Each patient who left before receiving a medical screening examination was flagged as a LWBS patient in the ED log. Triage did not count as medical screening.

2. The number of LWBS patients divided by the total number of visits gave a percentage of patients who left prior to a medical screening examination each day.

3. Daily LWBS rates were plotted in a control chart (p-chart [Figure 2.4]).

Figure 2.4

LWBS control chart

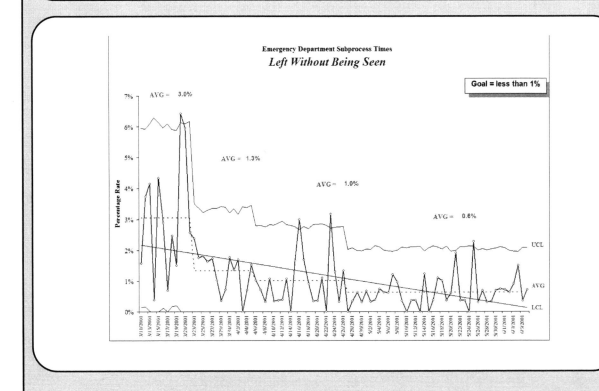

Case study (cont.)

4. Because the medical center believed that ED flow problems were related to the number of sick calls, such problems were plotted in a control chart (variance from staffing plan in staff-hours as well).

5. LWBS rates were plotted on the p-chart for the month prior to the study period.

6. As efforts were made to improve performance, daily data points were added to the chart. Three months' worth of data was reported to the improvement team each week and to key leadership each month. A monthly average also was calculated and added to the chart.

7. Improvements were swift and impressive. By establishing accountabilities for the triage team leader and implementing shortcuts to provider examinations, the average LWBS rate decreased to less than 1% and the fluctuations were muted. No one day had more than 3% of patients LWBS.

8. Satisfaction and billing increased as LWBS declined.

9. Monthly improvements to LWBS data were included in the hospital's patient flow scorecard (Figure 2.5).

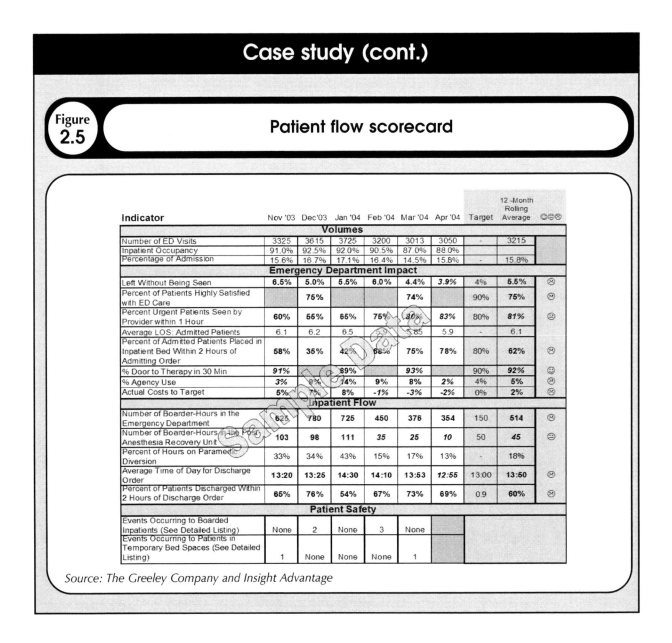

Case study (cont.)

Figure 2.5

Patient flow scorecard

Indicator	Nov '03	Dec'03	Jan '04	Feb '04	Mar '04	Apr '04	Target	12-Month Rolling Average	☺☺☺
Volumes									
Number of ED Visits	3325	3615	3725	3200	3013	3050	-	3215	
Inpatient Occupancy	91.0%	92.5%	92.0%	90.5%	87.0%	88.0%			
Percentage of Admission	15.6%	16.7%	17.1%	16.4%	14.5%	15.8%	-	15.8%	
Emergency Department Impact									
Left Without Being Seen	6.5%	5.0%	5.5%	6.0%	4.4%	3.9%	4%	5.5%	☹
Percent of Patients Highly Satisfied with ED Care		75%			74%		90%	75%	☹
Percent Urgent Patients Seen by Provider within 1 Hour	60%	55%	65%	75%	80%	83%	80%	81%	☺
Average LOS: Admitted Patients	6.1	6.2	6.5	5.9	5.85	5.9	-	6.1	
Percent of Admitted Patients Placed in Inpatient Bed Within 2 Hours of Admitting Order	58%	35%	42%	68%	75%	78%	80%	62%	☹
% Door to Therapy in 30 Min	91%		89%		93%		90%	92%	☺
% Agency Use	3%	8%	14%	9%	8%	2%	4%	5%	☹
Actual Costs to Target	5%	7%	8%	-1%	-3%	-2%	0%	2%	☹
Inpatient Flow									
Number of Boarder-Hours in the Emergency Department	625	780	725	450	376	354	150	514	☹
Number of Boarder-Hours in the Post Anesthesia Recovery Unit	103	98	111	35	25	10	50	45	☺
Percent of Hours on Paramedic Diversion	33%	34%	43%	15%	17%	13%	-	18%	
Average Time of Day for Discharge Order	13:20	13:25	14:30	14:10	13:53	12:55	13:00	13:60	☹
Percent of Patients Discharged Within 2 Hours of Discharge Order	65%	76%	54%	67%	73%	69%	0.9	60%	☹
Patient Safety									
Events Occurring to Boarded Inpatients (See Detailed Listing)	None	2	None	3	None				
Events Occurring to Patients in Temporary Bed Spaces (See Detailed Listing)	1	None	None	None	1				

Source: The Greeley Company and Insight Advantage

References

1. Institute of Medicine, *Crossing the Quality Chasm: A New Health System for the 21st Century,* March 2001.

2. The federal Emergency Medical Treatment and Active Labor Act. (See *www.cms.hhs.gov/providers/emtala/default.asp*)

CHAPTER THREE

Designing a new measure

Designing a new measure

We presented three questions for selecting an existing measure in **Chapter two:** *What are you trying to measure? How do you define the measure? How good is the measure?* These three questions also provide the framework for designing a new measure.

What are you trying to measure?

There are three steps involved in answering this question:

Step 1: Define how you will use the measure. To design a product or service that will succeed, you must understand the customer's needs. Therefore, start the process of designing a new measure by identifying the customer. Is the customer of this measure an emergency department (ED) staff member, manager, or researcher? Will hospital management or regulatory accreditation departments use the measure? How? Will the measure be publicly reported? Will you use the measure for learning and improvement, for judgment, for decision-making, for information, or for monitoring a change in condition?

Step 2: Define what entity you will measure. The entity could be a patient, specimen, object, or group of people. The measure you develop interacts with the entity you will measure, so you must understand the entity at this step in the design process.

Step 3: Identify the concept you will measure. To do so, use six dimensions recommended by the Institute of Medicine (IOM) report—safe, effective, patient-centered, timely, efficient, and equitable—as defined in **Chapter two.** Consider which of these dimensions you are measuring. In the ED setting, many (if not most) of the measure will focus on timeliness since the mission of the ED is medical screening and stabilization. The ultimate management and resolution of the problem is usually left to others, following discharge or after admission.

Some other dimensions measure cost, reliability, serviceability, aesthetics, flexibility, perception, or reputation. Appropriate here is measurement principle No. 2 in **Chapter one,** "Our theories determine what we measure." Get an opinion from an outside peer before determining which concepts to use.

How do you define the measure?

There are two steps involved in answering this question:

Step 1: Choose or develop a test method that relates to the concept. First, operationally define the concept you will measure. For example, if the concept is "weight of an ED patient," do you mean current measured weight or stated weight? What test methods are available for measuring the patient's weight? How will they interact with the patient? Should you select a weight scale built into the bed, an ambulatory scale, or a chair scale? The test method you choose or develop must operationally define the concepts into procedures or specifications that everyone can follow when measuring or discussing it.

There is often a tradeoff between feasibility and precision. For example, should you measure minutes, hours, days, or patients? Remember that you need a valid measure for all.

In your selection, consider cost, quality, and timing of the test method in your selection. For example, suppose the concept is "perception of the ED care." Instead of developing a written patient satisfaction survey, consider making videos of patients describing his or her experience at ED discharge or IP bed placement. The video may be faster and provide more important qualitative data for improvement to the ED.

Measurement principle No. 1 in **Chapter one** is "Change the method of measurement and you change the results," but what if no acceptable test method exists? Developing a new test method or modifying an existing one requires a prototype-testing phase to determine whether it measures the intended concept. A small-scale test of the prototype alongside an existing method might be appropriate.

Measurement principle No. 3 in **Chapter one** is "Choose scales and units of measure that optimize the learning of the user," but which scale (nominal, ordinal, ratio, or interval) will allow you to collect data related to the concept chosen in Step 3 of "What are you trying to measure?" What is the plan for collecting these data? How often and how many will you collect?

Standardized forms can ease the burden of collecting data and reduce systematic errors. Ask yourself: Can you capture the data electronically? What is the level of aggregation? How will you graphically display the result data? How will you analyze it? To answer these questions, understand the measure defined in Step 1 of "What are you trying to measure?" See **Chapter four** for more information about creating a data collection and reporting system.

Step 2: Do you need to establish criteria for judgment? When using the measure to make a judgment or a decision (such as determining regulatory or purchasing contractual requirements), you may need to convert it to an attribute that meets the criteria. Specifically, define what appropriate adherence to protocols mean. For example, what does on-time surgery mean? The attribute "on-time" would need a criterion to determine how much departure from the scheduled time the organization would tolerate and still consider the surgery to be on time. Also, consider issues related to uniformity of the attribute and sampling in establishing criteria for judgment.

How good is the measure?

There are two steps involved in answering this question:

Step 1: Determine the quality of your measure. The user of the measure must define a quality measure. Some characteristics that define a quality measure include the following: simple, inexpensive, accurate, precise, stable, reliable, and sensitive.

An accurate measure must have a high level of precision and no bias. Minimize the effect of variation of a measure by using good calibration practices to control bias and by repeating measurements to increase precision. For subjective measures, you can improve precision between and within rater reliability.

To assess the quality of the measure for any of the above quality characteristics, pilot-test the measures. Nearly all new measures will require some sort of revision after such pilot testing. Simple testing methods are found in **Appendix A** and for more detail, see *Planned Experimentation.*[1]

Step 2: Determine the relationship to other measures. No single measure will determine an overall performance of a complex system. A family of measures (system, suite, scorecard, dashboard) provides different perspectives for a more holistic understanding. Consider the following: What is the relationship of the new measure to another in the family? Plotting a scatter diagram of two measures (used on the same entity) reveals any relationships between them.

Case study

Choosing and developing boarder hours

A hospital was experiencing delays in patient admissions and wanted to establish a reliable and informative measure for tracking the efficiency of the inpatient bed placement process. It seemed that the problem had two causes: unnecessary delays in the admitting process and a lack of available inpatient beds.

Existing measures

Like many hospitals, this one had existing indicators to measure the admitting process, but staff were not entirely satisfied with the results. Existing measures did not seem to drive meaningful improvement:

  1. **Diversions hours:** The hospital tracked the number of hours paramedics were diverted from the ED due to "saturation." Although this measure was very important to the organization and the indicator was related to the admission process, diversion hours alone did not get to the issues:

     First, the decision to divert was relatively subjective—that is, managers and physicians would decide to divert based on different kinds of indications. Second, the number of diversion hours in part reflected the level of saturation of the entire paramedic

Case study (cont.)

catchment area. When one department started to divert, the others got a dispropor-
tionate share of new patients which sped up saturation for the next and the next and
the next. In other words, once one of their community peers was on diversion, the
rest quickly followed.

At best, monthly diversion hours were an indirect indicator of the inpatient admitting process and bed availability.

2. Average length of stay (LOS) for admitted patients: The ultimate goal of the
improvement effort was to decrease the LOS for ED patients—in other words, to
increase the functional capacity. The hospital decided to split the LOS into three
parts, as there were three fundamentally different back-end processes at work: LOS
for discharged patients, LOS for transferred patients, and LOS for admitted patients.

The LOS for admitted patients was 5.2 hours—not favorable when compared to the
LOS of other departments in the community. However, this LOS did not cleanly
point to the admitting process because other factors were involved, such as the efficiency of the medical screening process, the turnaround time of diagnostic suppliers
(radiology and laboratory), and the availability, response time, and speed of the
admitting practitioners.

Therefore, LOS for admitted patients, like diversion hours, was an important measure, but it was not exactly what they were looking for.

3. Bed turnaround times: The admitting department routinely tracked how long it took
to assign a bed after a request was made. Admitting was quite proud of its 30-
minute average.

The ED, however, did not find much meaning in the measure. A bed was often
assigned while it was still occupied by another patient, who had been discharged
according to the ADT (admission, discharge, and transfer) computer system but was

Case study (cont.)

still awaiting transportation, medications, medical equipment, final instructions from the nurse, or terminal cleaning by environmental services.

Therefore, the bed turnaround time meant that admitting's job was over, even though the patient remained in the hallway of the ED. It did not focus on the ED patients of delayed admissions.

4. Other measures: Similar considerations applied to other good but off-target indicators, including transportation turnaround time and environmental services bed turnaround time.

Developing the measure: Boarder hours

The Institute for Healthcare Improvement (IHI) focuses on boarder hours as a meaningful overarching indicator.

A boarder is defined as any patient who remains in the ED (or post-anesthesia care unit) beyond the ideal target for admission-processing time. Some hospitals feel the ideal target for admitting a patient, once the admitting order is written, should be one hour. Others have chosen two hours as the maximum time it should take to admit a patient. The hospital we worked with chose one-and-a-half hours as the trigger for boarder status. In other words, any patient who remained in the ED (or the post-anesthesia care unit) longer than one-and-a-half hours after the admission/transfer order was written was a boarder.

In this hospital, boarder hours are the total number of hours admitted inpatients remained in the ED beyond one-and-a-half hours.

Defining boarder hours

Monthly boarder hours equals total minutes to admission minus 90 minutes for each patient admitted. Negative boarder hours were ignored.

Case study (cont.)

The following logic was developed for use in a Microsoft Excel spreadsheet and could serve as the basis for programming these calculations into standard administrative reports for the appropriate database. The calculation is performed for each patient admitted through the ED or the operating room (OR).

Total boarder minutes: For each admitted patient, calculate the following: Minutes to admission minus 90. If minutes to admission < 90, total boarder minutes = 0

Total monthly boarder hours: For each month, the total boarder minutes for the month divided by 60

Adjusted monthly boarder hours (for 30-day month): Because the number of days (and, therefore, opportunities to board patients) varies from month to month adjust the data by adjusting the raw boarder hours.

Adjusted total monthly boarder hours = 30 divided by the number of days in the month.

For example:
February: 100 boarder hours * 30/28 = 107 adjusted monthly boarder hours
March: 100 boarder hours * 30/31 = 97 adjusted monthly boarder hours
April: 100 boarder hours * 30/30 = 100 adjusted monthly boarder hours

Defining minutes to admission

There is still one very important detail we had to work out: when to begin and when to end the admitting process clock. We decided on the following definition for minutes to admission (as used in the boarder hour calculation): time the patient was placed in an inpatient bed minus the time the order for admission was written.

Why not start the clock where there is existing data—that is, the time admitting is notified of the bed request? Because there were often problems with the timeliness of the bed

Case study (cont.)

request. The timely request for an inpatient bed was, from the patient's point of view, part of the process to be improved. If the measure did not include this segment of the process, then this segment would become invisible to the improvement effort.

Why not end the clock when a bed was assigned? As explained earlier, the bed was often assigned when it was not really available to the patient.

Data collection process

The hospital's ADT system had fields available for all the data points collected below, and routine reports were programmed for the manager and senior leaders. However, the same type of data collection can be collected manually (e.g., using a Microsoft Excel spreadsheet) until such information technology resources become available.

The unit clerk entered the time of the physician's admission order into the ADT system. She or he also enters the order for the inpatient bed. If the time of the admission order is not known to the clerk, the field is left blank. The computer has been programmed to calculate the following routine measures:

- ✓ Daily boarder hours (used for a control chart)
- ✓ Raw monthly boarder hours
- ✓ Adjusted monthly boarder hours (used on the leadership balanced scorecard)
- ✓ Data-capture rate: Time of order for admission (the inverse of the number of blank fields for time of admission order)
- ✓ Average time from admission order to time of order for admission

Therefore, if data capture was high (e.g., 90%) or the average time from admission order to bed request was low (e.g., less than 10 minutes), one could have confidence in the accuracy of the core leadership indicator, which is adjusted monthly boarder hours. On the other hand, if data capture was low or the interval between admission order and bed request was high, separate preliminary improvement efforts may be necessary.

In each of these measures, there are multiple options—and all could be correct. There-fore, you may devise different measures for different stakeholders. The goal of the effort will help guide which is the most appropriate method.[2]

As discussed, consider carefully how you will use the measure, what concepts and enti-ties you will measure, and what methods you will use. With each measure there are trade-offs between increasing precision and burden. However, do not sacrifice validity. Whether conducting clinical research or quality improvement, you need a valid measure that users of the data believe to be accurate. Many improvement and research projects fail because they lack such a measure.

The previous examples are all outcome measures but process measures (interventions) are also commonly used. Process measures examine how often we do what we ought to do. They are generally easier and less expensive to collect than outcome measures, although usually well received by caregivers, process outcomes are less important to patients, who typically care about outcomes.

Sample process measures for the ED

Literature from the Joint Commission on Accreditation of Healthcare Organizations' (JCAHO) *Specifications Manual for National Implementation of Hospital Core Measures* [3] suggests growing clinical evidence of an association between timely inpatient administration of antibiotics and improved outcome among pneumonia patients. Therefore, ED caregivers should provide the following:

1. Initial antibiotics within four hours of arrival
2. Blood cultures within 24 hours of arrival
3. Oxygenation assessment within 24 hours of arrival (pulse oximetry and ABGs)

To develop measures of quality of care for these actions, we needed to create specific def-initions. For example, how would we define "pneumonia" or "antibiotic"?

The numerator is defined as a patient who received any antibiotic during his or her ED stay, even if it did not meet the consensus guidelines.

References

1. R.D. Moen, T.W. Nolan, and L.P. Provost *Quality Improvement through Planned Experimentation, Second Edition* (New York: McGraw-Hill, 1999).

2. P.J. Pronovost, 2003.

3. *www.jcaho.org/pms/core+measures/information+on+final+specifications.htm.*

CHAPTER FOUR

Creating a data collection and reporting system

Creating a data collection and reporting system

When deciding on the data that you will collect, analyze, and report, ask yourself the following questions:

- ✓ How easy is it to collect the necessary information?
- ✓ Is the information consistently documented in the medical record?
- ✓ Is the information consistently captured in an administrative data set, such as the emergency department (ED) logging system?
- ✓ How accurate is the information collected?
- ✓ Who will do the data collection?
- ✓ Who will do the data analysis?
- ✓ Will data analysis methods be complex or simple?
- ✓ Will sampling be necessary?
- ✓ How will the data be displayed? Graphs? Scorecards?

This chapter addresses these and related issues.

Data collection

Many improvement efforts fail because a process (including the resources) to collect the data is not identified at the beginning. The data collection system and resources should be stable—that is, built to last indefinitely. Remember, most efforts to improve the ED require ongoing commitment and a stable data-reporting method. And in the real world of limited resources, this may mean that other existing data collection efforts are abandoned. Improving processes in the ED is often like reshaping a pillow—pushing a lump in on one side of the pillow often causes a new lump to appear on the opposite end. Therefore, as ED processes change (improve), it is not unusual to have corresponding processes change (deteriorate) implying the need for ongoing data collection to ensure continued stability.

Sampling

Sample size

To simplify data collection, take a random sample of what's being measured. The size of the sample you should take depends on how much sampling error can be tolerated (sampling error is the difference between the characteristics of the sample and the characteristics of the population being sampled)

For example, an ED wishes to measure the average time it takes to triage patients presenting to the department by sampling 70 records a week. How closely will the average calculated from the random sample approximate the average for all patients seen in the department?

For this example, suppose 1000 patients were triaged that week. In fact, the degree of the sampling error has little to do with whether you're sampling 70 out of 100, 70 out of 1000, or 70 out of 1,000,000. The sampling error for calculating an average based on a sample of "n" (70) patients is proportional to the standard deviation (SD) of the data measured (time to triage) divided by the square root of "n" (70). Assume that the SD for all triage times is 11 minutes so that

> ✓ for a sample of 70 records, the sampling error is 11 (SD) divided by the square root (sqrt) of 70 (sample size) or about 1.3 minutes
> ✓ for a sample of 30 records, the sampling error is 11/sqrt (30) = 2 minutes
> ✓ for a sample of 10 records, the sampling error is 11/sqrt (10) = 3.5 minutes

Consider an improvement team that wants to reduce the time to provider, measuring weekly performance over 25 weeks. How clearly they will be able to see any change will depend on the accuracy of the average triage times calculated, which will depend on the sample size. Let's assume that the real change is represented by the run chart in Figure 4.1.

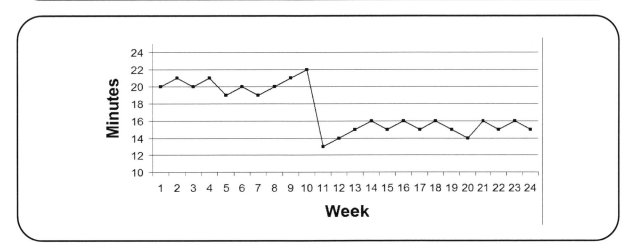

Figure 4.1 — Average triage time based on ALL triages

What happens when we sample using various sample sizes? Figure 4.2 shows how the same run chart might look given various sample sizes. Clearly, the chart at the top, based on a sample size of 70 records, gives a more accurate picture than the chart at the bottom, based on a sample size of 10.

Sample frequency

In the example above, the improvement team took its time (almost six months) to study the data and improve. However, most improvements are done more quickly. For example, what if you wanted to see what the day-by-day triage times were? You would measure more often (each day) to see the effects of the change. However, it may not be feasible to sample 70 charts per day just to get the data. Therefore, you could choose a smaller number. How few charts can be sampled to still see the change? That's a matter of judgment. Your team may choose to sample 20 records a day—a compromise between measurement nirvana and the reality of resource availability.

Figure 4.2 — Sample size run charts

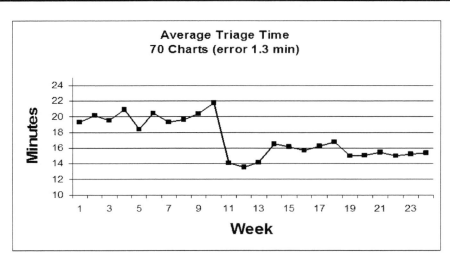

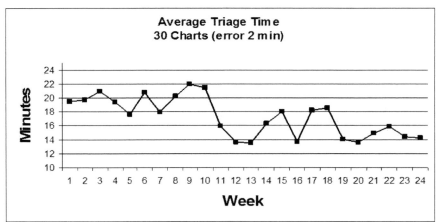

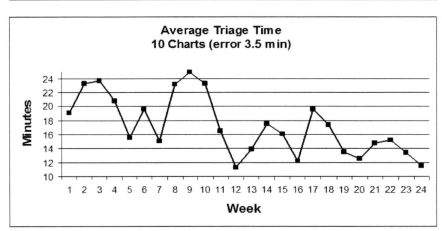

Consider the following questions when balancing the sampling decision:

✓ Is a concerted rapid improvement effort underway? Consider 15 random records a day.

✓ Is the process being measured to ensure stability? Consider 50 to 70 random records a month.

✓ Is the process not being looked at for change or stability? Don't bother measuring at all. See measurement principle No. 4 in **Chapter one,** "There is no need for measurement if the intended use is strictly historical." In other words, measurement should be viewed as a means to improve, not as an end in itself.

Other data collection issues

Forms

Some EDs use forms to collect information. Figure 4.3 is an example of a form used to collect information about transfers of patients to other facilities. This form has a good deal of utility for quality control purposes. The top part of this form is a checklist you can use to make sure all items are completed. The form also helps with supervision, so the manager will be able to check that all transfers were appropriately documented. An incidental purpose of the form is as a data collection tool. The bottom part of the form is used to collect data on transfers. In this case, the institution set thresholds for performance in four areas: timeliness of ambulance arrivals (one hour), the timing of nursing and physician notices (15 minutes prior to transport) and documentation of stability prior to transport.

Figure 4.3 — Interfacility transfer data collection tool

Emergency department

Quality control

Patient identification	
Date of transfer:	
Reason for transfer	❑ Unstable transfer/higher level of care ❑ Transfer after stabilization for continued hospitalization ❑ Transfer after stabilization for nursing facility care
Time of transfer order	
Time of acceptance by receiving facility	
Person accepting transfer on behalf of the receiving facility	
Time of acceptance of the receiving physician	
Name of accepting physician	
Time of ambulance notification	
Time of transfer	
Time of last documented physician evaluation/note	
Time of last nursing assessment note	
Documentation of transfer	❑ Consent for transfer (❑ N/A) ❑ Copies of medical records ❑ Transfer form complete

Process/Improvement information

Minutes from transfer order to ambulance response	Minutes: ❑ Greater than 1 hour
Minutes between last physician note and transfer	Minutes: ❑ Greater than 15 min
Time from last nursing notes to transfer	Minutes: ❑ Greater than 15 min
Was stability for transfer documented	❑ Yes ❑ No ❑ N/A

Displaying and analyzing the data

Run charts and control charts

The data in Figures 4.1 and 4.2 are examples of run charts. For an example of a true control chart (a run chart with control limits included) used to stimulate dramatic improvements at a client site a few years ago, see Figure 2.4 in **Chapter two.** The power of this type of display is that change is put into context and real change can be distinguished from the noise of natural variation.

Walter Shewhart, the father of control charts, introduced the concept that any variation in measure can be attributed to two types of causes:

1. *Common causes of variation:* Causes that are inherent in the process over time affect everyone working in the process, and affect all outcomes of the process.

2. *Special causes of variation:* Causes that are not part of the process all the time or do not affect everyone but arise because of specific circumstances.[1]

A process whose outcomes are affected only by common causes is called a stable process, or one that is in a state of statistical "control." "Stable" implies that the variation is predictable within bounds.

A process whose outcomes are affected by both common causes and special causes is called an unstable process. For an unstable process, the variation from one time period to the next is unpredictable. As special causes are identified and removed, the process becomes stable. You will recall in measurement principle No. 5 in **Chapter one,** that a measurement process must be stable for any measurement to have value.

A control chart is a statistical tool used to distinguish variation in a process due to either common or special causes. A control chart provides an operational definition of these concepts. This is accomplished by adding control limits to the run chart and a set of rules for special causes.

Control charts can be applied throughout any healthcare organization for a number of uses:

- To study variation in costs and revenue
- To assign responsibility for the improvement of a process
- To study variation in quality of outcome
- To determine whether a change is an improvement
- To determine when to adjust a process

Another example of a control chart for an overall patient satisfaction survey score is given in Figure 4.4. Control limits were recalculated when a distinct improvement in patient satisfaction occurred in May 2001. Shewhart and others developed a set of rules to determine when the process has changed and, thus, when control limits must be recalculated.

Figure 4.4

Control chart for survey score

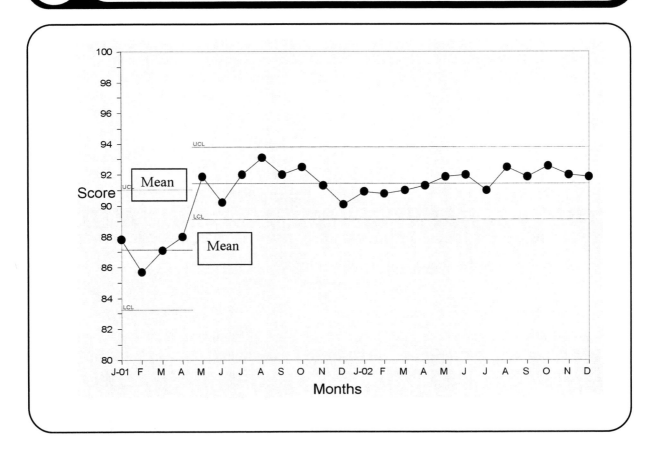

Other graphical displays

Edward Tufte, a world leader in graphic display of data, says a basic principle for a graphical display is "to communicate all the information contained in the data with the least amount of ink."[2] This principle is important because software products offer a variety of display options for data. Microsoft's Excel has several standard types of data display features: columns, bars, cylinder, cone, pyramids (all histograms), line, pie, scatter, area, doughnut, radar, surface, bubble, or stock. There is even a custom type option.

The second level of reporting systems is the graphical display of the data from a set of measures that define a system performance. A balanced set of measures (balanced scorecard) provides information from a variety of perspectives. These may include functional outcomes, clinical outcomes, financial measures, and patient satisfaction. The tabular display should allow the user to see all measures as a group. **Chapter five** goes into more detail about developing a balanced scorecard.

Another method for displaying multiple measures is using a spider diagram (or radar chart), such as that in Figure 4.5. The advantage of this format is that it provides a display of all measures in one graphic; the disadvantage is that it does not allow us to look at data over time.

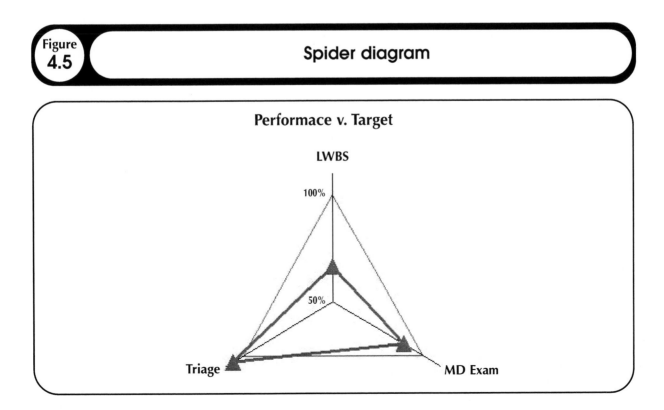

Figure 4.5

Spider diagram

Performace v. Target

As you improve in the areas of data collection and reporting, you enhance the ability of measures to become more effective and efficient. Figure 4.6 offers a checklist of measures, data collection, and graphical displays.

Table 4.1 on p. 49 outlines the steps involved in developing ED measures. Table 4.2 on p. 50 illustrates ED quality and performance measures with examples of hospital-wide measures in which the ED participates. Table 4.3 on p. 56 lists websites for indicator selection and development.

Figure 4.6	Checklist for measures

	YES	NO	Opportunity for improvement
1. Balance of measures is used			
• Uses 4-8 measures related to an overall aim			
• Includes outcome measures			
• Includes process measures			
• Includes other balancing measures			
2. Data collection procedures are defined and useful for improvement			
• Sampling is used			
• Stratification is used			
• Data is collected at least monthly (weekly or biweekly preferred)			
• Data collection is integrated into daily work routines			
• Data collection forms are used			
• Uses manual collection procedures instead of waiting for computer systems			
3. Improvement team focuses on usefulness, not perfection, of measures			
• Collects just enough data to see if changes to are leading to improvement			
• Uses qualitative data to supplement quantitative information			
• Improvements in the measures can be seen quickly			
4. Measures are used for learning			
• Measures are reviewed and interpreted by the entire team			
• Actions are directed at systems and processes, not people			
5. Data is displayed graphically			
• Clear and thorough labeling, including X and Y axis labels			
• Simple, with the least amount of ink			
• All measures can be viewed on one page			
• Includes context and important events			

Table 4.1: Steps to develop ED measures

Steps	Considerations
1. Conduct literature review	Computer search engines are a wonderful source of potential ED indicators. Both The Joint Commission on Accreditation of Healthcare Organizations (JCAHO) and the Centers for Medicare & Medicaid Services (CMS) have active indicator development processes. Being up to date is essential, especially since comparing your performance with available national norms is helpful. (See Table 4.3 for helpful Web sites.)
2. Find out what's important to executive leadership	There are a number of processes that take place in the ED that are, or should be, important to senior business leaders (e.g., admission rate, paramedic diversions, patient satisfaction). There is another set of indicators that are targeted for improvement by clinical leaders (e.g., care of patients with congestive heart failure, care of patients with acute myocardial infarction, timeliness of the first dose of antibiotics for pneumonia patients, etc.). Unless the ED measures "connect" with executive leadership, there will be little impetus for improvement.
3. Select specific outcomes or care processes to monitor	A dashboard of important indicators should be selected that 1) address key goals of the organization (e.g., clinical excellence, satisfaction and efficiency) and 2) have appropriate levels of sponsorship. Remember that the reliability of data is also important (see **Chapter five**).
4. Select pilot indicators	By looking at the data available to the department and the resources already dedicated to quality control, the ED should be able to focus on a few vital indicators of performance. Define the measure very carefully, including numerator, denominator, and unambiguous data source.
5. Evaluate the reliability/ validity of the data	Start collecting the data and see how often it is reliably entered into the medical record or other registration/logging system. Also, be careful of differing definitions given by other departments.
6. Pilot test the measures	Just because a measure is developed and defined does not mean it can or should be collected. Put aside plenty of time to test the measures, including a realistic idea of how many resources it will take to collect and analyze the data over time.

Table 4.2: ED quality and performance measures

Note: Departments nationwide are typically involved in measuring two "families" of clinical indicators:

1. Measures of ED and hospital operations, which are primarily process indicators
2. Measures of larger clinical processes in which the ED is only a part (e.g., the care of patients with acute myocardial infarction)

Quality measure	Comment
Examples of hospital-wide measures in which the ED participates	
Risk-adjusted mortality rates (e.g., acute myocardial infarction [AMI] mortality rates)	These rates only are useful when defined identically to other hospitals in the same data cohort. For example, the state of California publishes risk adjusted AMI mortality rates. Data specification are set by the benchmarking entity. Normally, mortality rates are meaningless unless risk-adjusted. Collect demographic information and detailed information about condition upon presentation. Extensive chart abstraction is normally required.
JCAHO ORYX core indicators	
Care of patients with myocardial infarction	
Time to thrombolysis	Mean time from arrival to thrombolysis for patients with AMI
Time to percutaneous coronary intervention (PCI)	Mean time from arrival to PCI for patients with AMI
Aspirin upon arrival (AMI)	AMI patients without contraindication who receive aspirin within 24 hours of arrival
Beta blocker at arrival	AMI patients without contraindication who receive a beta blocker within 24 hours of arrival

Table 4.2: ED quality and performance measures (cont.)

Care of patients with pneumonia	
Timeliness of administration of the first dose of antibiotics for patients with pneumonia	The time from arrival to first dose of antibiotics is measured for all patients with pneumonia. It is then reported as the percent receiving the first dose within eight hours and the percent receiving the first dose within four hours.
Surgical infections	
Timing of prophylactic pre-surgical antibiotics.	The proportion of surgical patients who have prophylactic antibiotics administered within one hour prior to surgery (within two hours prior to surgery if vancomycin or a fluoroquinolone is administered)
Selection of prophylactic pre-surgical antibiotics	The proportion of surgical patients who have prophylactic antibiotics administered which meet current selection guidelines
Other hospital-wide indictors that include ED performance	
Patient satisfaction rates	These rates are measured and collected using a method that will allow comparisons in the cohort
Falls	Per hospital definition
Sedation/anesthesia-related complications	Per hospital definition
Use of restraint	Per hospital definition
Appropriateness of admissions	Per hospital definition
Medication errors	Per hospital definition
Retention rates	Sometimes used for JCAHO staffing effectiveness indicators

Table 4.2: ED quality and performance measures (cont.)

Registry utilization	Sometimes used for JCAHO staffing effectiveness indicators
Nursing hours per visit	Sometimes used for JCAHO staffing effectiveness indicators
Failure to rescue	This is a relatively new indicator made prominent by HealthGrades' 2004 report on medical error.[3]
ED-focused indicators	
Discrepancy rate in x-ray interpretation between ED and radiology	Numerator: Number of discrepancies between the emergency medicine impression and the impression by radiology. Denominator: Number of x-rays read by emergency medicine and referred to radiology for "over reading."
Appropriateness of admissions	Appropriateness rates are usually focused on such diagnoses as chest pain and other problem prone DRGs.
Timeliness of ED care	
Timeliness of triage	Number of minutes from time of arrival to time of triage. True time of arrival is preferred but rarely collected. Time of first contact with department personnel is typically used as a substitute. Time of triage end is preferred over time of triage initiation. However, time of triage end is not always consistently recorded in the medical record. Reporting should be percentage of patients where time of arrival to time of triage is less than 15 minutes. (If either true time of arrival or time of triage end are used, consider expanding the threshold to 20 minutes.) Also consider a secondary threshold to report outliers, such as percentage of patients triaged 60 minutes or more after arrival.

Table 4.2: ED quality and performance measures (cont.)

Timeliness of physician examination	Number of minutes from time of arrival to time of emergency provider examination (physician, nurse practitioner, etc.). If a reliable triage system is used, consider reporting the timeliness of bed placement by triage category. The urgent or middle category of a five-tier triage system will provide most EDs with a lot of useful data. Consider the routine use of a scatter diagram with time of day on the category, or x-axis, and the number of minutes from arrival to provider examination on the value, or y-axis. This will show the severity of mid-afternoon backlogs (see Figure 4.8).
Timeliness of bed placement	Number of minutes from time of arrival to time of ED bed placement. Time of physician examination (above) is the preferred measure. However, time of bed placement may be a more reliable measure depending on the data capture and accuracy of provider examination time.
Timeliness of consultation response	Number of minutes from emergency medicine request for consultation to the time the consultant is in the patient's room. Exclusions: consultations from specialties that are not on the call panel. This measure should be reported by specialty. Some documentation processes require nursing to record consultant-at-bedside time, since the consultant often documents the time of dictation instead of time at bedside.
Timeliness of admission process	Median/mean time from request for an inpatient bed to the time the patient is on the inpatient unit.
Boarder hours	Patients are defined boarders if they remain in the ED for greater than an hour after a request for an inpatient bed has been transmitted to the responsible party. Some hospitals may wish to define a boarder more liberally, giving one and a half to two hours for inpatient bed placement. Calculation: See **Chapter three.**

Table 4.2: ED quality and performance measures (cont.)

Laboratory turnaround time	Turnaround times for the clinical laboratory should be measured for defined sets of frequently used studies (e.g., chemistries, urinalysis, cardiac studies, etc.).
	Turnaround time is defined as the number of minutes between the time the laboratory study was ordered and the time the result was posted to the ED chart. (Note: The lab's definition of turnaround time may be different.)
	Rather than mean or median time, a performance guarantee should be negotiated between the ED and the laboratory. The percentage of studies meeting this threshold should be reported. A secondary trigger should also be set to look at distribution. For example, 1) percent of cardiac studies posted to chart within 30 minutes of order and 2) number greater the 60 minutes from order.
Radiology turnaround time	Separate turnaround times should be collected for routine x-rays, CT scans, MRI studies, and ultrasounds.
	Turnaround time is defined as the number of minutes between the time the imaging study was ordered and the time the interpretation was posted to the ED chart.
	Use the same reporting method use for lab studies—a double-tiered threshold.
Treadmill turnaround time	Turnaround time is defined as the number of minutes between the time the treadmill electrocardiogram was ordered and the time the interpretation was posted to the ED chart.
Utilization of diagnostic studies	Physician-specific rates of diagnostic testing should be calculated for selected laboratory and imaging studies
Physician productivity	The number of patients seen per hour should be reported on a physician-specific basis. Include physician assistants and other provider categories in the productivity report.

Table 4.2: ED quality and performance measures (cont.)

Rate of patients who leave without being seen (LWBS)	Numerator: The number of patients recorded as having LWBS. Denominator: Number of visits. Daily rates should be collected and the monthly mean reported. If the LWBS rate is greater than 5% or patient satisfaction is low, daily LWBS rates should be displayed on a run chart.
Timeliness of analgesia	Percentage of patients who are given pain-relieving treatment within 30 minutes of the initial report of pain. Note: Reporting the median time may also be useful. Exclusions and relieving treatment should be carefully defined.
Monthly saturation diversion hours	Number of hours the ED diverts paramedic traffic due to ED saturation (insufficient space or staff). It is helpful to display diversion hours as a proportion of the total number of hours in the month (on average there are 730 hours per month).
Bed density	Numerator: Number of patients discharged (does not include the number of patients who LWBS). Denominator: Number of staffed ED beds; excludes hallway beds.
Length of stay (LOS) for discharged patients	Number of minutes from time of arrival to time of discharge for patients whose disposition is *home*.
LOS for admitted patients	Number of minutes from time of arrival to time of discharge for patients whose disposition is *admit*.
LOS for transferred patients	Number of minutes from time of arrival to time of discharge for patients whose disposition is *transfer*.

Table 4.3: Web sites for indicator selection and development

The pace of change in the third millennium is incredible. Leading this rapid transformation is the ever-evolving information super highway: the internet. Therefore, please remember that the Web sites referenced here will evolve; new outstanding sites will emerge and old sites will disappear or become irrelevant. Please view this list as a starting point. Also remember your best ally in researching indicators and benchmark information is a good internet search engine. We like Google™.

Organization and Web site	Description
Institute for Healthcare Improvement (IHI) *www.ihi.org/IHI*	IHI has a robust site with white papers, books, and other information, both for free and for sale, relating to patient safety and quality.
Joint Commission on Accreditation of Healthcare Organizations (JCAHO) *www.jcaho.org*	Among the many features at the JCAHO Web site are a number of links that relate to ORYX indicators.
National Quality Forum (NQF) *www.qualityforum.org*	The NQF is a not-for-profit organization created as a public-private partnership to develop and implement a national set of quality measures and report them. NQF has developed a rigorous set of quality of care measures that are widely accepted as a national measure set. It has become the first general set of performance measures. Among the robust list of products is the 2003 *National Voluntary Consensus Standards for Hospital Care: An Initial Performance Measure Set.*
RAND *www.rand.org*	Rand is a nonprofit institution that helps improve policy, and decision-making through research and analysis. Rand has an entire section on healthcare with a robust array of articles and other documents on ambulatory and hospital quality, including suggested indicators.
Agency for Healthcare Research and Quality (AHRQ) *www.ahrq.gov*	AHRQ, a part of the U.S. Department of Health and Human Services, is the agency charged with supporting research designed to improve the quality of healthcare, reduce its cost, improve patient safety, decrease medical errors, and broaden access to essential services. Indicators and guidelines are among the very deep resources available on the site.

Ways to measure process times

In emergency medicine, the timeliness of care directly relates to satisfaction, quality of care, patient safety, efficiency, and profitability. It is not surprising then that most meaningful measures of ED performance are related to time intervals, such as timeliness of thrombolytics therapy, timeliness of analgesia, and timeliness of patient bed placement.

The way times are reported can make a big difference in how performance appears. Here are some things to consider when selecting the way to measure time intervals:

Mean: The mean, which we normally think of as the average (although median and mode are averages as well), is often useful and is the most common measure of performance. However, average alone is rarely useful in getting an idea of performance. We find average process times to be most useful when trended over time.

Median: Most prefer to use the median rather than mean time when dealing with averages. The median (half are above and half are below) reduces distortion due to outliers.

Maximum: Looking at the maximum time can be a useful supplement to the average time (median).

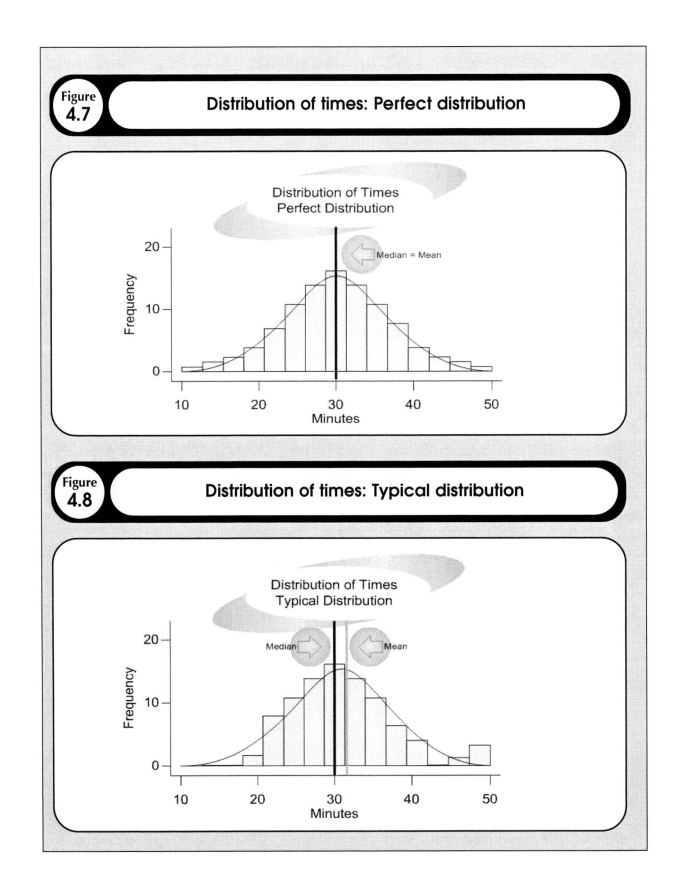

If there is a performance expectation involved with a time threshold (e.g., patients will be triaged within 15 minutes of arrival, or critical laboratory values will be reported within 30 minutes of the lab order), we often find it useful to report percentage of time the threshold was met—for example, percentage of patients triaged within 15 minutes.

At other times, descriptive statistics are less important than every data point. For example, in Figure 4.9, the actual distribution of times to triage by time of day can be more informative than any average. The target of 15 minutes (dark horizontal line) is met most of the time. However, quality, safety, and satisfaction issues arise over the occasional hour wait for triage.

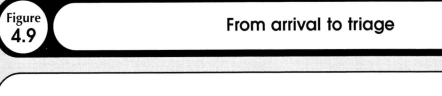

Figure 4.9 — **From arrival to triage**

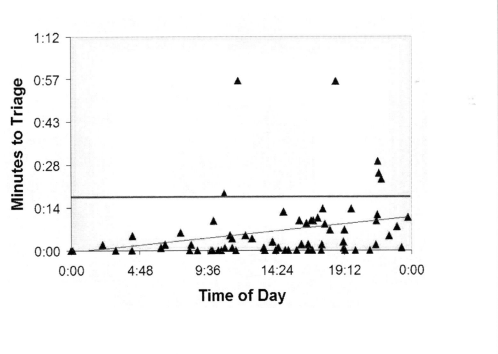

Source: The Greeley Company and Insight Advantage.

References

1. W.A. Shewhart, *Control of Quality of Manufactured Product* (Milwaukee: *American Society of Quality Control,* 1931) (reprinted 1980).

2. E.R. Tufte, *The Visual Display of Quantitative Information, Second Edition,* (Graphics Press, 2003).

3. HealthGrades Quality Study: *Patient Safety in American Hospitals* (July 2004) *www.healthgrades.com/media/english/pdf/HG_Patient_Safety_Study_Final.pdf* (accessed October 2004).

Seven steps to uncorking the ED bottleneck by deploying effective scorecards

Seven steps to uncorking the ED bottleneck by deploying effective scorecards

Focusing leadership's attention

The solutions to the most troubling and visible emergency department (ED) problems are beyond the ED's direct control. To solve these problems, EDs must work with executive leaders to influence the performance of other hospital departments and medical disciplines.

The ED is an important "front door" to the hospital. Its mission is to stabilize and plan an appropriate disposition for whatever patients come its way. The stability and smoothness of its operations depend heavily on the pre-hospital care system and the efficiency of the hospital's inpatient service. In other words, its problems are sometimes symptoms of the dysfunction of others.

Of course, the ED can do much on its own to improve performance, but the larger problems (such as paramedic diversions, extended ED lengths of stay, and missed admissions) though visible in the ED, are controlled by others. For example, to provide for a swift and appropriate medical screening examination, the laboratory, the imaging department, and the cardiology service must serve the ED efficiently. To avoid paramedic diversions, inpatient service must provide an appropriate location for patients who require admissions. We believe that the best way to focus leadership's attention on the right monitors to affect these issues is to develop a leadership scorecard that addresses the overall flow of the patient: from the door of the ED to the wheelchair home, following an inpatient admission.

This chapter describes the different kinds of scorecards and dashboards used across the nation and brings together the concepts introduced in **Chapters 1–4** that enable the ED manager and emergency medicine chief to champion a cross-departmental, interdisciplinary effort aimed at improving patient satisfaction, clinical quality, and operational efficiency.

The power of the scorecard

Scorecards and dashboards are among the latest trends, and for good reason. They are fundamental management tools used very effectively elsewhere in the business world and they've only just begun to grow into the world of clinical operations.

Physician and nurse managers, like managers in all businesses, are used to being judged based on scorecard results. Executive leaders use traditional scorecards to hold managers accountable for the basic performance of their department (Figure 5.1). They typically focus on performance to budget (revenue v. expenditures) and productivity measures (nursing hours per visit; patients per physician per hour) and because these measures are important to executive leadership, they are very important to management. They truly drive performance, sometimes in unexpected and non-productive ways. Note: The subject of budgetary disincentives to smooth patient flow is discussed in the authors' book, *Solving Emergency Department Overcrowding: Successful Approaches to a Chronic Problem.*[1]

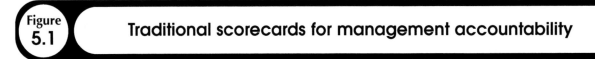

Figure 5.1   Traditional scorecards for management accountability

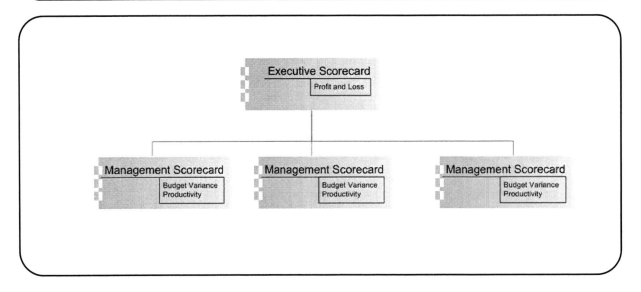

Cross-departmental and interdisciplinary scorecards can be equally effective in driving performance, if properly designed and implemented (Figure 5.2). But the ED manager and emergency medicine chief will have to overcome a number of hurdles if they plan to drive the adoption of such a tool. Such hurdles include the following:

✓ The issues measured on the scorecard must be important to executive hospital and medical staff leadership

✓ Other departments involved in the measures (e.g., inpatient nursing, laboratory, imaging, and environmental services) must agree to have their success or failure judged, in part, by scorecard performance

✓ Some scorecard measures exist but are in the "territory" of other services, such as case management

✓ Some scorecard measures do not exist or are inaccurate and resources must be found (diverted from other tasks) to capture the data

✓ The scorecards must be created routinely and reported to leadership, which requires resources (usually within the quality improvement department)

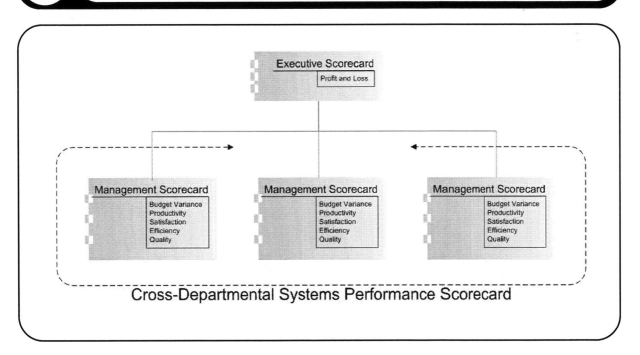

Figure 5.2

Balanced scorecard—Clinical operations

But it's not all bad news:

> ✓ Using a scorecard to address these issues will help the institution thrive: profits will increase as quality, efficiency, and satisfaction are enhanced. (You may find an ally in the chief financial officer!)
>
> ✓ The Joint Commission on Accreditation of Healthcare Organizations (JCAHO) requires leaders and "supplier departments" to measure, assess, and improve indicators of patient flow (standard LD.3.15, effective January 1, 2005).

Real time v. retrospective scorecards

Some institutions have developed real-time scorecards, many of which evolved from bed tracking/management tools. These scorecards or dashboards are used to anticipate "kinks" or shortages in the patient flow system and are used to facilitate bed management "huddles" at the beginning of each day. These tools try to anticipate the impact of both the OR schedule and the current census so that nurse and ancillary staffing can be planned and physician resources can be mustered to "clear the decks."

This technology is working well in a number of institutions. Although it is easier if the hospital has an automated patient tracking system, scorecards can be implemented based on essentially manual processes, when necessary. (For a broader discussion of flow tracking please refer to *Solving Emergency Department Overcrowding*.[1]) Here we will discuss leadership accountability for ongoing performance.

Seven steps to scorecard nirvana

Where do you go now that you understand the wisdom of developing a cross-departmental scorecard? Odds are that, if you're still reading this chapter, you will be involved in the scorecard development process. To that end, we've segmented the process into seven discrete steps, which you should take one at a time.

Step 1: Find out what's truly important to executive leadership

If it's important to you and you have control over all the moving parts, you and your department can effect change. If you don't have control over all the moving parts—as will be the case with the most important issues that impact the ED—it is essential that you gain the support and acceptance (not merely the tolerance) of the right level of executive leadership.

"But wait," you say. "I've been working with other departments for years without involving executive leadership. It seems to work fine."

True and false. ED department managers have learned over the years how to influence and work with other departments to bring about change without involving executive leadership. But it isn't working well at all. The reason is simple: No matter how much the other department may want to help out the ED, they will focus on that for which their boss holds them accountable. If you don't do what your boss expects, either you or your boss are likely to change positions soon.

"But getting executive leadership support is almost impossible," you complain. True. That is why we've outlined these seven steps. If the issues you face are important enough, executive leadership will support them. However, you must approach the right level of executive leadership—neither too high nor too low (see step 5)—and you must do your homework.

Before you even begin, however, determine where the issues of importance fall within the hierarchy of leadership concerns:

> ✓ Is leadership in financial turnaround? If so, emphasize measures that will enhance revenue or decrease costs.
> ✓ Is leadership committed to improving customer/patient satisfaction? If so, take the time to determine the elements of satisfaction at risk (e.g., time to analgesia for patients presenting with complaints of pain) and consider focusing on process steps likely to enhance satisfaction.
> ✓ Is leadership troubled by lost admissions due to paramedic diversions? If so, emphasize improvements that will enhance the functional capacity of the unit.
> ✓ Is leadership committed to demonstrating the highest possible quality of care? If so, emphasize measures of quality that will be visible to the Leapfrog Group, the JCAHO, or the Centers for Medicare & Medicaid Services.

If you don't connect with one or more strategic goals of executive leadership, you're unlikely to gain their support.

Some have used a matrix approach to align potential indicators with strategic goals. Figure 5.3 is an example from an institution where the overarching concerns were satisfaction, clinical excellence, efficiency, and compliance. This matrix connects each proposed measure to one or more of the strategic goals. It also addresses the departments and disciplines involved and, therefore, the level of sponsorship necessary (step 5).

Figure 5.3 — Indicator matrix

Indicator	Priority improvement area				Operational focus				Sponsorship			
	Satisfaction	Clinical excellence	Efficiency	Compliance	Professional staff	Nursing	Diagnostic/ Therapeutic services	Support services	Vice president	Chief executive officer	Medical executive committee	Professional staff committee
Time to ED provider examination	●	●	●	●	●	●				●	●	
LWBS rate	●	●	●		●	●				●	●	
ED LOS by disposition	●	●	●	●	●	●	●	●		●	●	
Admit processing time	●	●	●			●		●		●		
Consultation response time	●	●	●		●					●	●	
ED boarder hours	●	●	●	●	●	●	●	●		●	●	
Inpatient LOS			●		●	●	●	●		●	●	
Supplier TAT			●				●	●		●		
Nursing report processing time	●	●	●			●			●			

Step 2: Assess existing indicators

Once you've identified the issues that are important to leadership, begin to look for indicators that other departments already use to measure these processes. It is very likely that anything very important to leadership has already been measured somehow.

✓ Look at the "bed board" or other dashboard tools to see if there are the some measures that will address monthly performance report cards.

✓ Check with case management to see what leadership already receives in terms of case mix and length of stay.

✓ Meet with the chief financial officer to learn about the performance reports that are already scrutinized.

✓ Look at the hospital's quality plan to see what other departments are monitoring.

Step 3: Find the gaps

Keep a list of all existing indicators and see how many of them address the overall matrix you have in mind. Identify the gaps in broad strokes. Ask yourself the following questions:

✓ Are supplier (radiology, laboratory, environmental services) turnaround times measured? If so, are they internally defined, or are they defined in terms of the ultimate customer? For example, laboratory turnaround times should not be from accession to report but from order to placement in the medical record.

✓ Is there a reliable measure of boarder hours?

✓ Are departmental indicators accurate?

✓ Is data collection stable and ongoing?

✓ Are existing indicators credible?

Step 4: Evaluate candidate indicators to fill the gaps

News flash: There are only so many data collection and analysis resources available. Therefore, any new indicator you propose will likely supplant an existing indicator. Sometimes hospitals make the mistake of thinking they can do it all, and instead of supplanting existing indicators, new measures are heaped on top of the old with the effect of paralyzing data collection/aggregation efforts. However, when new workloads are added to existing resources, something will be supplanted whether we wish to acknowledge it or not.

It is therefore important to scope out each proposed indicator carefully. Otherwise, when you shop for executive sponsorship, you will be delayed (or perhaps unsuccessful) because you haven't been thorough and you haven't considered the consequences/tradeoffs inherent to the new indicator.

Figure 5.4 is a worksheet devised by a hospital to help executive leadership examine indicators as they are proposed. Using a process like this will help you think through the implications of developing the measure. The example is for the indicator "boarder hours." The hospital in question developed this worksheet to facilitate this exercise.

Figure 5.4

Indicator worksheet

Indicator Name: **ED and UCC Boarder Hours**

Name of Scorecard(s) on Which Indicator will be displayed

Leadership Patient Flow Scorecard

Improvement Priority	Satisfaction	Clinical Excellence	Efficiency	Compliance
Degree of Relationship	Medium	High	High	Low
Explain (unless no relationship)	Patients/families tend to be less satisfied with extended ED stays	Inpatient care units are a safer location for the care of inpatients.	Boarded inpatients decrease nursing and physician productivity and decrease functional capacity.	This indicator is one possible element of the leadership patient flow scorecard required by JCAHO.

<u>Disciplines</u> contributing to the process or system measured by this indicator	<u>Departments</u> contributing to the process or system measured by this indicator	
✓ Nursing ✓ Administrative and Support	✓ Emergency Department ✓ Central UCC ✓ Virginai Mason Hospital	✓ Admitting Department ✓ Inpatient Nursing ✓ Housekeeping

Longevity of the Issue Studied

[X] Indefinite/ Ongoing   [ ] **Time Limited.** Issue will disappear on   because

Data Element(s)	Data Source(s)	Calculation
1. Time Admitting Order is Complete 2. Time Patient is Placed in an Inpatient Bed	✓ Medical record ✓ ADT System	#1 minus #2 (minutes between order and admission) less 90 minutes (acceptable admit process time) for each admitted patients

Are all data elements constantly collected / recorded?	No
Are all data elements accurate?	No
Who will collect and prepare the data for reporting?	ED / UCC Manager
Is this an existing indicator (already in use)?	No

Comments

Minor changes are necessary to the ED / UCC computer system to redefine fields. Routine reports must also be programmed and management trained.

The accuracy and consistency of data collection requires improvement.

Contact: Name, Title.   **Date of Submittal:**   **Status:**

Figure 5.4

Indicator worksheet (cont.)

Instructions

✓ Please be brief. Try to fit all information on one page.
✓ Use the tab key to move from field to field.
✓ For questions call: #####
✓ Email completed for to NNNNNN.

Approval of the Quality Improvement Committee Required

The Hospital Quality Committee ("Committee") is responsible for focusing the attention and resources of the hospital to promote the swift and lasting improvement of high risk, high volume or problem prone processes. To achieve the necessary focus, the Committee applies criteria (see below) to select the indicators and analysis techniques commensurate with the data collection, information analysis and resource allocation capabilities of the institution. It is therefore the policy of the hospital that all improvement indicators, including the collection, analysis and reporting of these indicators, receive prior Committee approval.

Exception 1—Implementation Testing. Whenever a clinical or operational process or system is new or significantly changed (e.g. new computer system, new policy, new registration process, revised patient identification system, revised triage system) the person or group responsible for the new or improved process is expected to monitor the system / process to assure its stability. This monitoring is usually done only during implantation. Such monitoring may be as complex as data driven pilot testing or as simple as validating staff understanding of the new process by spot checking performance on various shifts. This type of data collection and testing does not require the improvement of the Quality Improvement Committee unless it is expected to extend beyond the process implementation phase.

> **Example:** A root cause analysis is performed following an adverse clinical event. A change in the patient identification system is made to address the root cause of the event. The managers responsible for the patient identification process make improvements and then monitor implementation through observational studies. They continue the data collection until they are assured that staff are consistently following the policy. **Approval for this type of data collection and monitoring is NOT required.**

Exception 2—Management Control/Quality Control. Departmental leaders are expected to establish mechanisms to assure high risk or problem prone processes are carried out consistently and accurately. Examples of such management tools include the maintenance and review of refrigerator logs, review of all restraint documentation to make sure all applicable information is recorded, maintaining logs of testing for activity levels of disinfectants, etc. Which measures are established, how they are collected and who reviews them is left to the discretion of the departmental leadership. Such management / quality control does not require Committee approval.

However, Committee approval is necessary should Implementation Testing or Management / Quality Control point to an aspect of hospital operations that requires broad-based or long term improvement. For example, Implementation Testing of a new patient identification system may point out the need to focus on improving communication techniques; or, routine Management / Quality Control monitoring of restraint documentation may highlight the need to improve the use of alternatives to physical restraint.

Figure 5.4

Indicator worksheet (cont.)

Approval of Scorecards / Data Displays

The Committee will not normally review and approve an indicator without the context in which the data is displayed. It prefers to approve each scorecard / data display rather than just the component indicators.

The criteria guiding the Committee's consideration of the proposed scorecard / data display are the same as those guiding the consideration of individual indicators (see below).

Criteria to Guide the Consideration of Proposed Indicators

1. **Alignment with Improvement Priorities.** Hospital leadership has adopted the following priorities for improvement:

    a. **Satisfaction:** Maximized patient, customer, staff and physician satisfaction is a fundamental goal of the hospital and the Cooperative.

    b. **Clinical Excellence:** We are committed to the continuous improvement of clinical quality and patient safety.

    c. **Efficiency:** There is a fundamental connection between efficiency, quality and safety. Furthermore, efficient systems preserve the resources of the organization. Normally, indicators that measure efficiency alone should be displayed alongside related measures of quality or safety (when such measures are available).

    d. **Compliance:** Some measures are specifically required by an accrediting or regulating body. Although compliance considerations are important, the Committee expects that all indicators, including those implemented in the name of a regulation or standard, also address satisfaction, quality or efficiency.

2. **Departments and Disciplines Involved in the Process.** To judge whether the sponsorship level for an indicator set is appropriate, the Committee needs to know which departments and disciplines are involved in the process.

3. **Sponsoring Persons or Groups.** Indicators or scorecards/displays will not be approved unless an appropriate person or group within the leadership structure has agreed to receive reports, allocate resources for data collection and analysis, and take actions aimed at improving performance.

    The sponsoring person or group should have oversight responsibility for the performance of all departments and disciplines involved in the process measured.

Step 5: Get the right level of executive sponsorship

How do you choose the right level of sponsorship? Simple: Identify where in the organization responsibility for the performance of all players in the process under study come together. Don't go to the higher level, as that will only complicate matters. For example, in Figure 5.5 we developed a simplified organization chart supposing that the ED wants to monitor and improve the application of the nursing triage scale. We also assume that this process is completely under the control of the ED nursing manager, who should therefore be the sponsor. Transferring sponsorship to the next highest level will make improvements unnecessarily complicated.

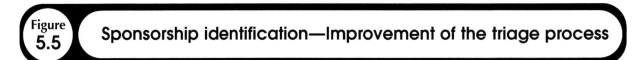

Figure 5.5 Sponsorship identification—Improvement of the triage process

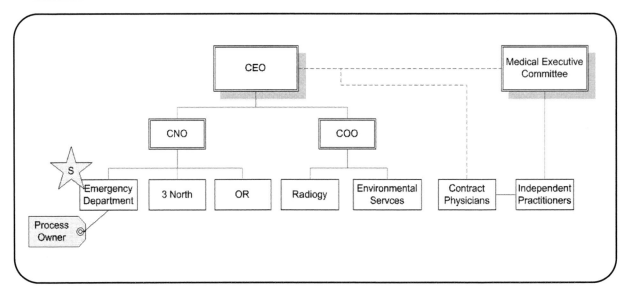

Figure 5.6 supposes that the nursing report process is to be measured and improved for 3 North, a telemetry unit. The only departments involved are 3 North and the ED. Accountability for these departments converged under the chief nursing officer (CNO), therefore the CNO should sponsor this monitoring/improvement.

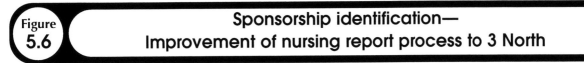

Figure 5.6

Sponsorship identification—
Improvement of nursing report process to 3 North

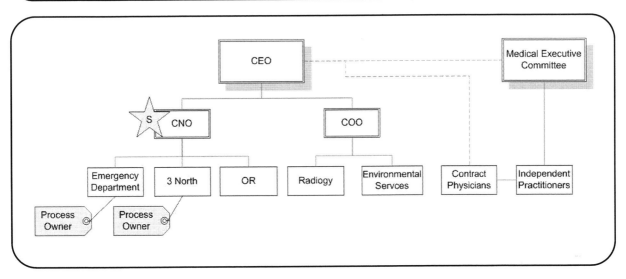

What about improving physician productivity? The CEO is responsible for contracting
with the ED physicians and therefore should be the sponsor of the project (Figure 5.7)
The next proposed indicator involves consultant response time (Figure 5.8) and must, of
course, involve the medical executive committee.

Figure 5.7

Sponsorship identification—
Improvement of physician productivity in the ED

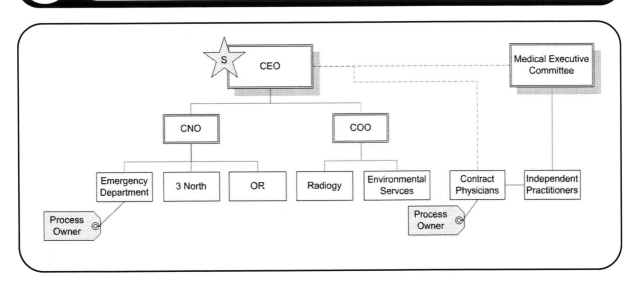

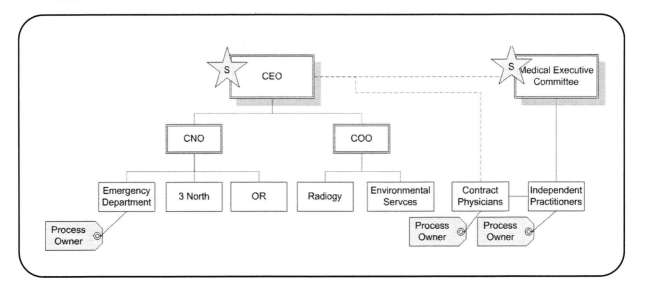

Figure 5.8

**Sponsorship identification—
Improvement of consultant response time to the ED**

The final example (Figure 5.9) considers radiology turnaround times. This type of indicator is typically negotiated between the nursing and radiology managers during hallway conversations. When the time is not taken to obtain the right level of sponsorship, however, performance may be measured but will rarely improve.

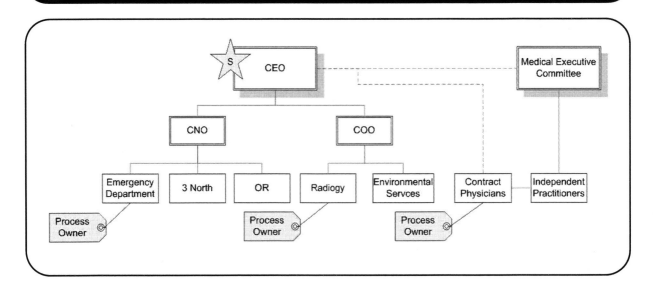

Figure 5.9

**Sponsorship identification—
Improvement of radiology turnaround time**

Before moving on, we should prepare you for one last difficulty. Getting managers to agree to measure things like radiology turnaround times is relatively easy because everyone is interested in doing their best for the patients and empathizes with their peers, however, getting managers to agree on a measure in front of the appropriate sponsors will be difficult, because everyone knows that actual improvements will become part of their boss's evaluation system. The manager will want to be especially certain that the measure is accurate and that performance is truly achievable. And that is not easy.

Step 6: Set two performance targets for each indicator

Improvement is indeed continuous, but for the purposes of developing a scorecard, performance targets should be identified.

We recommend two thresholds: one for acceptable performance and one for exceptional performance. Exceptional performance should be rewarded. Less than acceptable performance should trigger feedback to all involved parties and, perhaps, a formal improvement effort.

For example, the acceptable time to analgesia may be less than 35 minutes. An exceptional time may be set at less than 25 minutes. Therefore, three ranges are established: exceptional, acceptable, and less than acceptable. In setting these or any other targets, take current performance into account. If current performance is one hour, you may choose to set the acceptable time at 45 minutes, at least for the interim. Setting unachievable targets demoralizes the players and diminishes the credibility of the scorecard process.

Step 7: Measure, report, and improve

Now that the scorecard is in place, it is time to truly improve. Implementing improvements are the easiest and most satisfying parts of the process.

Figure 5.10 is a sample scorecard used by one of our clients. Note that it is all on one page and uses emoticons (happy and sad faces) and shades for ease of interpretation.

Figure 5.10

Sample scorecard

Indicator	Nov '03	Dec'03	Jan '04	Feb '04	Mar '04	Apr '04	Target	12-Month Rolling Average	☺☺☹
Volumes									
Number of ED Visits	3325	3615	3725	3200	3013	3050	-	3215	
Inpatient Occupancy	91.0%	92.5%	92.0%	90.5%	87.0%	88.0%			
Percentage of Admission	15.6%	16.7%	17.1%	16.4%	14.5%	15.8%	-	15.8%	
Emergency Department Impact									
Left Without Being Seen	6.5%	5.0%	5.5%	6.0%	4.4%	3.9%	4%	5.5%	☹
Percent of Patients Highly Satisfied with ED Care		75%			74%		90%	75%	☹
Percent Urgent Patients Seen by Provider within 1 Hour	60%	55%	65%	75%	80%	83%	80%	81%	☺
Average LOS: Admitted Patients	6.1	6.2	6.5	5.9	5.85	5.9	-	6.1	
Percent of Admitted Patients Placed in Inpatient Bed Within 2 Hours of Admitting Order	58%	35%	42%	68%	75%	78%	80%	62%	☹
% Door to Therapy in 30 Min	91%		89%		93%		90%	92%	☺
% Agency Use	3%	0%	14%	9%	8%	2%	4%	5%	☹
Actual Costs to Target	5%	7%	8%	-1%	-3%	-2%	0%	2%	☹
Inpatient Flow									
Number of Boarder-Hours in the Emergency Department	625	780	725	450	376	354	150	514	☹
Number of Boarder-Hours in the Post Anesthesia Recovery Unit	103	98	111	35	25	10	50	45	☺
Percent of Hours on Paramedic Diversion	33%	34%	43%	15%	17%	13%	-	18%	
Average Time of Day for Discharge Order	13:20	13:25	14:30	14:10	13:53	12:55	13:00	13:50	☹
Percent of Patients Discharged Within 2 Hours of Discharge Order	65%	76%	54%	67%	73%	69%	0.9	60%	☹
Patient Safety									
Events Occurring to Boarded Inpatients (See Detailed Listing)	None	2	None	3	None				
Events Occurring to Patients in Temporary Bed Spaces (See Detailed Listing)	1	None	None	None	1				

Source: The Greeley Company and InSight Advantage

Reference

1. D. Pete and B. Pate, *Solving Emergency Department Overcrowding: Successful Approaches to a Chronic Problem* (Marblehead, MA: HCPro, Inc., 2003).

CHAPTER SIX

Understand the pros and cons of improvement methods

Understand the pros and cons of improvement methods

Many hospitals are trying to implement Six Sigma, Lean Thinking, or other improvement models borrowed from manufacturing and other industries. Each of these systems works magnificently to improve quality, efficiency, and the financial bottom line. But remember that all of these improvement models are fueled by data, data, data. So don't miss the improvement wave by sitting on your data; have it "at the ready" and use it to advocate for hospital-wide improvements that will make life easier—for you, for the ED, for the institution, and for the patient.

The recent focus of hospital C-Suites (the executive suite, where the chief executive officer, chief financial officer, and chief "you-name-it" officer sit) on Six Sigma and Lean Thinking has reminded them that there is more to improving hospital finances than cutting budgets. These new, trendy management models emphasize that improving efficiency (Lean Thinking) and decreasing defects (Six Sigma) is good for patients, good for staff, good for physicians, and wonderful for the financial health of the organization.

This chapter will define what we mean some of the buzz words, and help you choose from the "flavors of the month." It will give you plenty of information to answer with knowledge and assurance the next time the CEO asks "So, should we go with Six Sigma consulting?" You will be able to

✓ influence leadership decision making
✓ strategize your participation in the improvement process
✓ make sure that, whatever system is chosen, problems in the ED won't be moved to the back burner

The more things change, the more they remain the same

Are these new systems really different than what we've done in the past? It depends who you ask:

✓ Those who advocate for the new system will tell you it's revolutionary. "It will transform the way you do business overnight," they might say. "It's totally different from whatever you've done before."

✓ Skeptics will have a "been there, done that" look in their eyes. They've heard it all before. And because whatever happened before didn't work, they believe this new system won't work either. "I've got better things to do with my time," they'll think.

We fall somewhere in the middle—a little more toward the advocate than the skeptic. These new systems really do work, at least in other industries. Some hospitals and physician practices are also beginning to show impressive results. So if someone from the quality department or the C-suite gives you the word that a consultant is coming next week to begin training in Six Sigma, Lean Thinking, or any of the others, smile and say "Fantastic. We've heard that system is incredible for addressing ED issues. Let me know what I can do to help!" The new system could fizzle even if you support it. However, it you turn your back on it, you lose no matter what.

In our view, these new systems are "evolutionary" rather than "revolutionary." They are all based on the same sound management principles made popular by legendary quality experts Shewhart, Edwards Deming, and Joseph Juran. They all share a few fundamental principles:

✓ You cannot improve what you do not measure. All these systems rely on good, solid process data.

✓ Data must be analyzed carefully; otherwise, they can mislead as easily as they guide.

✓ The best person to design the details of a better process is the person closest to the process (front-line physicians and staff members).

✓ Quality should be defined in terms of the "customer" (usually the customer is the patient).

✓ Executive leadership must advocate for and drive improvements.

✓ Improvement efforts must be supported by adequate educational and analytical resources.

✓ The institution should establish a set improvement model, such as Plan, Do, Study, Act (Shewhart) or Diagnose, Measure, Assess, Implement, Control (Six Sigma) see Figure 6.1.

Figure 6.1 Improvement cycles

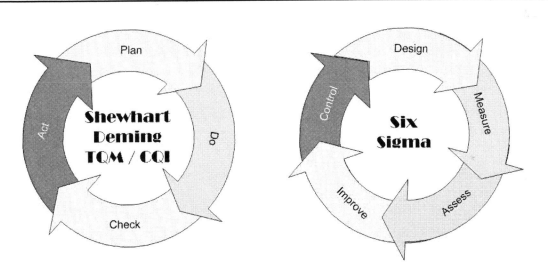

Most systems address improvement as a continuous, repeating cycle. The Shewhart Cycle is shown in this illustration along with the Six Sigma DMAIC process.

The tools are not the system

When we look at improvement systems, we often get distracted by their most visible aspect: the tools.

- ✓ In TQM or CQI, we became acquainted with control charts, Pareto diagrams (Figure 6.2), and Ishikawa (cause and effect) diagrams (Figure 6.3).
- ✓ In Six Sigma, you're likely to hear folks talk about multiple regression analysis or failure mode effects analyses.
- ✓ In Lean Thinking, we spend time on "tick marking."

But these tools are not really what makes Lean Thinking different from Six Sigma different from TQM. In fact, all of these systems can use all of these tools and others.

Figure 6.2

Pareto analysis

Factors contributing to a problem are counted with the most frequent displayed on the left, the next most frequent issue next, and so on. It is a very effective tool for focusing improvement efforts. But of course, you have to have the data before you can do the analysis.

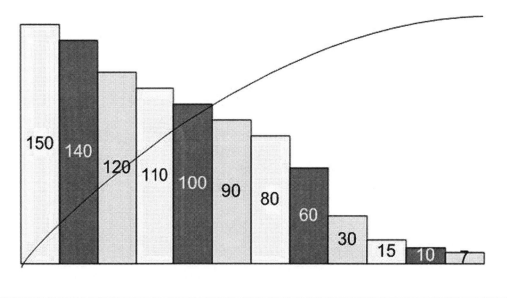

Figure 6.3 — Cause and effect or Ishikawa diagram

This tool is commonly used to identify the different factors that influence a process. The main spine of the fish (horizontal, from left to right) represents the process itself. Write the outcome or product at the nose. The four arrows intersecting the main spine represent important influences on the process. For example, most processes are influenced by supplies, human resources, physical environment, and customer expectations. Various components of these important process influencers are "arrowed" in from the side.

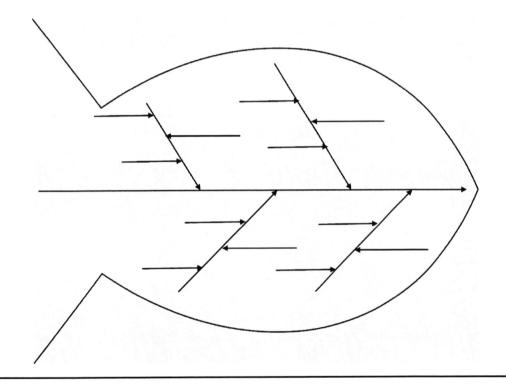

Understanding data: A core management competency

Data analysis techniques are fundamental to managing complex systems in the third millennium. If you're not familiar with these tools, become familiar with them now. (**Note:** A quick resource for management data analysis is *Understanding Variation: The Key to Managing Chaos* by Donald J. Wheeler.)[1]

No one expects a busy ED manager or emergency medicine physician to be a spreadsheet wizard or to throw a control chart together on the back of a lunch napkin. But it is essential that you know enough about data analysis to (a) recognize bologna when you see it and (b) know how you need to collect and analyze your own data to drive improvements. Give yourself this self test:

1. Do you know how to tell whether a spike in your LWBS rate is significant or just part of routine variation?
2. Do you know with precision when a change you've implemented really improved performance?
3. Do you know the best tool for studying your wait times as the day progresses?
4. Can you select the best way of studying your chart flow systems to uncover the key candidates for improvement?
5. Are you able to give specific instructions to staff as to how your door-to-provider times are to be analyzed?
6. Do you know the best way to see whether you've made a true dent in falls prevention?

If you are unsure of ANY of the questions above, consider spending some time studying business data analysis tools . . . soon.

Culture change

To be effective, all of these approaches usually require a significant culture change within the institution. They require complete alignment of the hospital and its staff, from the executive suite to the bed side, from the medical staff to environmental services, from diagnostic imaging to plant engineering.

Will it work in healthcare?

All of these models were developed for other industries and adapted for healthcare. Is healthcare really that different? Why shouldn't other industry approaches also work in healthcare? Good questions—we don't quite know the answers.

Definitions and distinctions

Now that we've talked about how these systems are the same, let's review how they are different.

Total Quality Management

Total Quality Management (TQM) has been around for decades. One of the most common and visible tools of TQM are our old friends "statistical process control" and the "control chart." Deming is normally thought of as the father of TQM, with his remarkable success in Japan in the 1950s, but his star is surrounded by a galaxy of influential predecessors (such as Walter Shewhart), contemporaries (such as Juran), and successors (such as Philip Crosby and Kaoru Ishikawa).

TQM is a way of managing, not a quality control process driven by staff. Yes, it's based in data, but it uses quality planning, quality improvement, and quality control as ways of managing a business.

Six Sigma

Six Sigma is one of the next evolutionary steps after TQM. The Six Sigma (6σ) process is aimed at reducing defects. The name says it all: Sigma (σ) is the Greek letter used by statisticians to mean "standard deviation." Most processes are pretty accurate, functioning at three sigma with 93.3% accuracy (see Figure 6.4). However, at three sigma there are more than 66 thousand defects per million opportunities. The goal of a Six Sigma company is near perfection: 3.4 defects per million opportunities, or 99.9997% perfect.

Figure 6.4 — **Sigma**

Most processes function with a 6.7% defect rate, or three sigma (3σ), with more than 66,000 defects per million opportunities. The goal is the near perfection performance of 6σ, with only 3.4 defects per million opportunities.

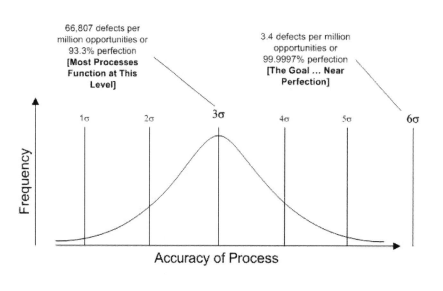

66,807 defects per million opportunities or 93.3% perfection **[Most Processes Function at This Level]**

3.4 defects per million opportunities or 99.9997% perfection **[The Goal ... Near Perfection]**

Here are a few things that make the Six Sigma model stick out:

✓ It is aimed at reducing errors (defects).

✓ All six sigma projects must have a demonstrable return to the financial bottom line.

✓ It is highly structured, with a cluster of tools linked to each step.

✓ It is resource intensive:

   o Project teams normally meet once a week.

   o There are "experts in training" on the team. These are called Green Belts and White Belts.

   o A full-time expert is assigned to the team (the expert usually facilitates up to four teams at once). This is a Black Belt.

   o The Black Belt is mentored and supported by an external consultant: a Master Black Belt.

   o The team demands the focus and attention of an internal leadership champion.

  o The team reports regularly to senior/executive leadership.

  ✓ The team and the organization receive training, training, training.

Pro

  ✓ The tools and the structure work (the success rate in other industries is about 80%).

Cons

  ✓ It is very expensive.

  ✓ Not all important healthcare processes have existing data for use with the 6σ toolbox.

  ✓ There is not always a demonstrable, short-term relationship between improved quality and financial performance.

Lean Thinking

Lean Thinking grew in the 1980s and, like Six Sigma, has become a very popular and successful approach for all sorts of businesses. However, a Lean Thinking project takes a slightly different tack: it focuses on making a system or process "leaner" or simpler, with fewer steps. Specifically, it focuses on reducing the non-value-added steps in a multi-step process. These steps are called "muda," the Japanese word for waste.

Case study

Lean Thinking: Finding the wheelchair

A friend of ours used Lean Thinking tools to help one hospital solve delays in the transportation of discharged patients. A two-hour wait was not uncommon between the time transportation was requested and the time the patient left the room.

The hospital's leadership identified this as a priority for improvement because of the "upstream" impacts of this downstream delay. Excessive delays in discharge (due, in part, to delays in transportation) meant delays in making the bed available for the next admission.

This meant that inpatients were kept in the ED, filling up the hallways to the point that new patients brought in by paramedics had to be kept in the paramedic ambulance that

Case study (cont.)

brought them. The ambulance was therefore not available for the next run. There were actually times in this community when all available paramedic ambulances were parked outside this hospital's ED and were therefore not available to respond to the next 911 call.

Like Six Sigma, Lean Thinking must make a connection with the institution's financial bottom line. The connection in this case was easy: The cost of delayed informal transports added to the costs of missed admissions and extended lengths of stay.

The quality and safety impacts of this issue were likewise self-evident.

Creating the team

Like all good quality projects, the Lean Thinking improvement team included the people actually doing the work (transporters), other staff involved in the discharge process (nurses, ward clerks, etc.), and the nursing director (who was also the leadership sponsor). Because of the impact on the ED, the ED nurse manager was also part of the team—she also wanted to learn about the process, thinking it might be useful in streamlining her triage and bed placement processes.

Working the problem

Figures 6.5 and 6.6 illustrate a simplified flow chart of the discharge transportation process and a sample of how value-added and non-value-added steps were identified. This was the first part of the team's work and was facilitated by an external consultant.

Case study (cont.)

Figure 6.5 — Tracking the wheelchair hunt

Lean Thinking projects typically start with a diagram of the process under study. It then uses a "tick mark" process to see how long it actually takes to perform each step in the process.

Process of Transporting a Patient from their Room to the Front Door during Discharge

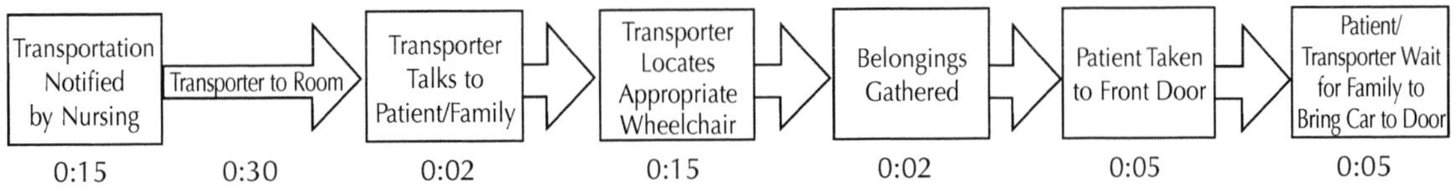

Transportation Notified by Nursing	Transporter to Room	Transporter Talks to Patient/Family	Transporter Locates Appropriate Wheelchair	Belongings Gathered	Patient Taken to Front Door	Patient/ Transporter Wait for Family to Bring Car to Door
0:15	0:30	0:02	0:15	0:02	0:05	0:05

Case study (cont.)

Figure 6.6

Reducing non-value-added steps

Steps are separated into two categories: those that give direct value to the customer and those that do not. The aim of Lean Thinking is to eliminate or reduce the time taken for those steps without value to the customer.

Before Improvement

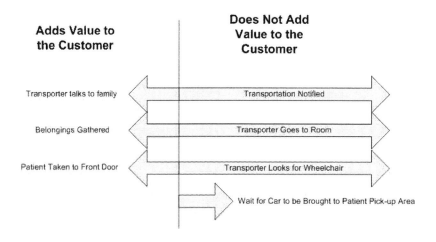

After Improvement

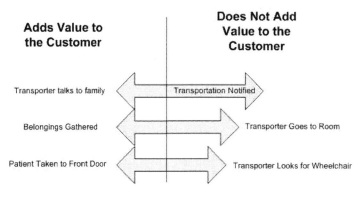

Case study (cont.)

Reducing the time for finding the wheelchair

Lean Thinking tools can be quite powerful when applied to the right problem. How this team found a key flaw in the transportation process illustrates this point nicely. Lean Thinking improvement processes can reduce the time it takes to perform non-value-added steps. To see a difference, however, it is necessary to collect the current time it takes to do the process.

For example, the time it takes a transporter to find a wheelchair is definitely not a valuable expense of time from the patient's point of view. Therefore, the hospital's team set out to measure how long it really took to perform this step.

Two members of the team were assigned to follow each transporter as he or she went about his or her daily tasks. In Lean Thinking, these types of observations were very structured and focused. One person followed the transporter to list each successive activity performed. A second person noted the time it took to perform each task. The team was amazed when they gathered at the end of the day to analyze their findings. Consider the following observation to illustrate:

- ✓ Transporter assigned to take John Doe from room 101 to the front door for discharge
- ✓ Travel to room 101 (0:02)
- ✓ Interaction with patient and family (0:01)
- ✓ Travel to elevator lobby of first floor to find available wheelchair (unsuccessful) (0:01)
- ✓ Travel to elevator lobby of second floor to find available wheelchair (successful) (0:01)
- ✓ Travel to room 101 with wheelchair (0:02)
- ✓ Attempt to transfer patient to wheelchair (unsuccessful: wheelchair too small) (0:05)
- ✓ Return wheelchair to elevator lobby (0:01)

Case study (cont.)

✓ Travel to elevator lobby of first floor to find available "big boy" wheelchair (unsuccessful) (0:01)

✓ Respond to page from supervisor (0:02)

✓ Travel to elevator lobby of second floor to find available "big boy" wheelchair (unsuccessful) (0:02)

✓ Travel to elevator lobby of third floor to find available "big boy" wheelchair (unsuccessful) (0:01)

✓ Travel to elevator lobby of fourth floor to find available "big boy" wheelchair (unsuccessful) (0:02)

✓ Travel to elevator lobby of fifth floor to find available "big boy" wheelchair (successful!) (0:01)

✓ Travel to room 101 with wheelchair (0:02)

✓ Transfer patient (0:03)

✓ Respond to page from supervisor (0:02)

✓ Travel to front door (0:02)

✓ Wait for car to be pulled around (0:05)

✓ Transfer patient to car (0:05)

✓ Return wheelchair to elevator lobby (0:01)

✓ Transporter available for next assignment

(Total time: Approximately 40 minutes. During that 40 minutes, five other unmet requests for transportation were received.)

In response to these observations, the hospital standardized where wheelchairs were kept and bought two more oversized models. More important, the Lean Thinking approach and tools made a significant difference to the patient discharge transportation process.

Influencing leadership's decision

How does one influence such a decision? After all, the ED does not control the entire institution.

The best way is to continue to connect quality and safety problems with finances and drive the point home in the executive suite:

✓ Show the connection between the LWBS rate and patient satisfaction
✓ Show the connection between patient satisfaction, walk-in urgent care, and revenue
✓ Show the lost admissions due to diversion hours
✓ Show the loss of functional capacity due to excessive lengths of stay
✓ Remind administration that the JCAHO now requires demonstrable improvements

Most of these issues will require actions by a number of departments, not just the emergency department. The connection between finances, quality, and compliance should help influence administration that a system—any system—is necessary, and that it should look first at the impact on the ED.

Which system works best for ED problems?

Any system, if properly implemented, will work just fine. It just takes the commitment and focus of leadership to make it succeed.

Reference

1. Donald J. Wheeler, *Understanding Variation: The Key to Managing Chaos, 2nd ed* (SPC Press, 1999).

APPENDIX A

Evaluating measurement systems

Evaluating measurement systems

Selected measures provide windows through which we are able to observe the performance of a process or system. If those windows do not provide predictable, consistent views, it is difficult to make intelligent decisions about what actions to take. As the saying goes, "A man with one watch knows what time it is. A man with two watches is never sure."

Figure A.1 illustrates that we are always looking through a window when studying outcomes of a process or system. Variation in the measured value can come from two sources:

1. The variation of the system or process being measured (due to people, methods, materials, equipment, environment, or measurement)

2. The variation contributed by the measurement process

Figure A.1 **Measurement as a process**

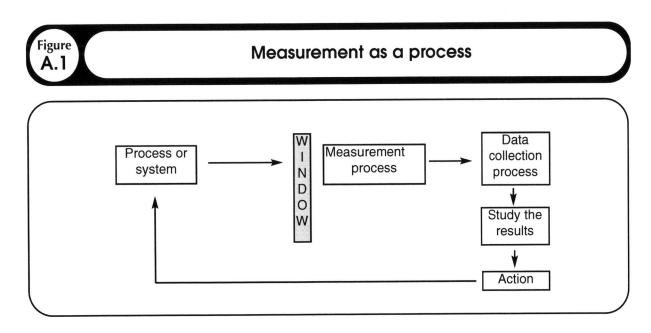

Variation in the measurement process can be due to the following sources:

- **Data collection** (recording, form, rounding error, error in data entry, error in wording)

- **Materials** (type, size, preparation, stability)

- **Equipment** (complexity, training required, mechanical, electronic, computer interface)

- **Method** (complexity, standards, calibration procedure, subjective procedure)

- **People** (training, fear, peer pressure, interpretation, openness, subjective method)

- **Environment** (cleanliness, noise, temperature, humidity, barometric pressure)

If more than one of the above sources of variation exist in the measurement process, it will be difficult from the data to learn about a single cause of variation. Understand the capability of the measurement system in order to advance knowledge of our processes and systems.

Studying the quality of a measure

In selecting an existing measure or designing a new measure as described in this book, you were presented with the question "How good is the measure?" Quality of a measure can be defined as the following:

Accuracy	Reliability	Simplicity
Bias	Repeatability	Speed
Cost	Reproducibility	Stability
Limit of detection	Robustness/ruggedness	Validity
Precision	Sensitivity	

Definitions for these terms are given in the glossary. "Validity," the extent to which a measure reflects the desired attribute of interest, has been used throughout this book.

There is no true value for a quantity. Accepted values (or accepted standards) may be legal values, consensus values, agreement values, or values obtained from a standard (or reference) method. Accepted standard values will always be subject to modification or obsolescence.

The amount of accuracy required for a test method depends on how the results of measurement are to be used. A measurement process with an acceptable level of accuracy is called accurate.

Accuracy, bias, and precision were defined in **Chapter two.** The concepts are illustrated in Figure A.2.

Only one of the four measurement processes illustrated in Figure A.2 has a useful level of precision and bias, and can thus be considered accurate. In healthcare, accuracy generally equates "unbiased" with "accurate" rather than defining "accurate" as both "unbiased" and "precise."

The stability of a measurement process is very important (measurement principle No. 5 in **Chapter one**). The measurement process must be in a state of statistical control in order for the precision or bias to have any meaning. The stability of the bias is much more important than the actual magnitude of the bias, because a known bias can be corrected through calibration. Control charts for accuracy and precision of a measurement process can be used to determine stability.

Precision for classification data

Precision for classification data can be evaluated by repeating the measurement process on the same samples or objects of measurement. If the measurement relies heavily on a person's judgment, the repeat measures should be made in a blind (unknown to the observer) manner. If two different observers or inspectors measure the same objects, the reproducibility of the measurement process can be determined.

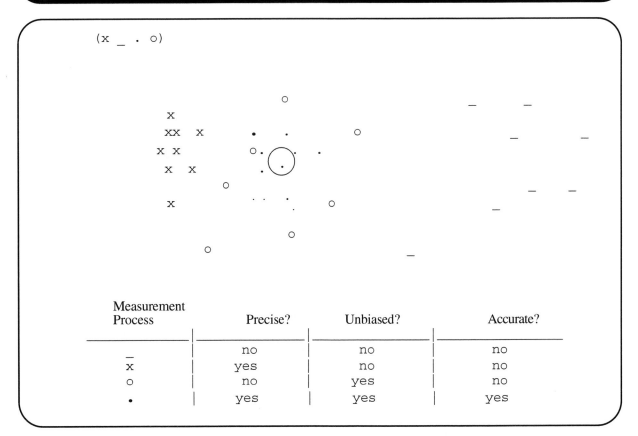

Figure A.2 — Illustration of precision, bias, and accuracy with four measurement process

Figure A.3 summarizes the results of a study to evaluate the precision of a classification measurement based on the examination of x-rays by two interns. Fifty x-rays were selected for the study. Approximately two-thirds of the x-rays were from patients later determined to have disease "A," and the remainder were from patients with disease "B." The x-rays were coded and independently evaluated by the two interns. The x-rays were then reordered and again submitted to each of the interns as a second group of 50 x-rays.

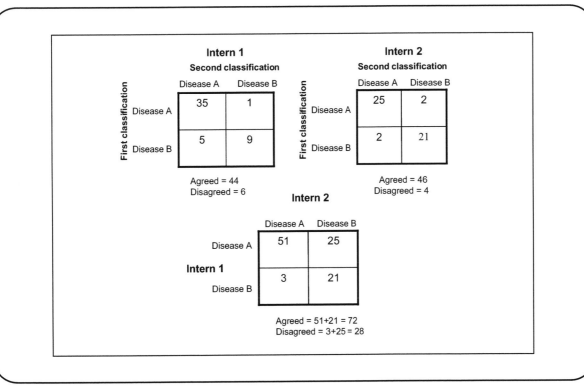

Figure A.3 — Measurement process evaluation

You can evaluate the repeatability of the measurement process by comparing the first classification to the second classification for each intern. A very precise measurement method would show agreement between the two evaluations. There were 44 (out of 50) agreements for intern 1, and 46 agreements for intern 2. The overall repeatability of the measurement method could be described as "90% agreement on repeated evaluations."

The reproducibility of the measurement process in this example is determined by comparing the results of the two interns on the 100 x-rays (two sets of the same 50 x-rays). They agreed on 72 of the evaluations and disagreed on 28. The reproducibility of the measurement method could be described as "72% agreement between interns on the same x-rays."

The best way to evaluate and describe the precision of a measurement method that gives classification data is generally a two-way table that compares repeated uses of the measurement method. Rank data with two levels (e.g., conforming/nonconforming parts) could be analyzed in a similar manner.

Measurement discrimination and rounding of numbers

Another issue that often arises when using a measurement process is the rounding off of quantitative data as it is recorded. This becomes an important issue in improvement because many of the available methods are based on studying the variation in data. For example, rounding off numbers can affect the observed variation. Rounding off data becomes important whenever the smallest unit of measurement exceeds the process standard deviation.

The paper by A.L. Propst[1] suggests that the smallest increment that can be read using the measurement system should not exceed one-tenth of the total process variation. D.S. Holmes and A.E. Mergen[2] use information theory methodology to evaluate the importance of the increment of measure (or unit of calibration). They conclude that an instrument should have units that are smaller than 30% of the process standard deviation.

Follow a general guideline to be sure that the way the measurements are being recorded gives adequate discrimination. Specifically, record data to as many decimal places as the measurement process will allow. The data can then be rounded for different uses as needed. When rounding of the data is necessary, record the data to at least one more decimal than the order of magnitude of the process standard deviation (e.g., __ = 0.03, round the data to thousandths).

More guidance on evaluating measurement systems

Improving a measurement process is no different than improving a process for production or service. You can use planned experimentation[3] to identify important sources of variation in the measurement process.

References

1. A.L. Propst (1989–90). "Verification of a Shop Floor Measurement System." *Quality Engineering* Vol. 2, no. 1 pp. 1–12.
2. D.S. Holmes and A.E. Mergen (1991–92). "A Discussion of the Unit of Calibration Required for a Gauge." *Quality Engineering,* Vol. 4, no. 1 pp. 1–7.
3. R.D. Moen, T.W. Nolan, and L.P. Provost (1999). *Quality Improvement through Planned Experimentation, Second Edition,* (McGraw-Hill, New York.)

APPENDIX B

Additional case studies

Additional case studies

Case study #1: First dose of antibiotics

A hospital-wide improvement team wanted to address the timing of the first dose of antibiotics for patients admitted with pneumonia. This issue came to the forefront in part because the hospital had selected the pneumonia indicators from among the Joint Commission on Accreditation on Healthcare Organizations (JCAHO) ORYX core indicator sets. The literature supports administering antibiotics within four hours of the arrival of patients admitted with pneumonia. JCAHO's pneumonia indicators measure, among other things, the percent of pneumonia patients who are given the first doses of an antibiotic within four hours and eight hours of arrival.

The team recognized that the JCAHO had established a reporting specification for this and related indicators. However, the team also weighed the option of reporting performance as a continuous variable: the mean or median time to antibiotic administration. The advantage of using a continuous measure was that the team could pick various thresholds and identify whether administering antibiotics in less than four hours was associated with improved outcomes.

In writing the study specifications, the team decided to follow the JCAHO's lead. Included in the study were patients admitted as inpatients with

- ICD-9-CM Principal Diagnosis Code of pneumonia

OR

- ICD-9-CM Principal Diagnosis Code of septicemia AND ICD-9-CM Other Diagnosis Codes of pneumonia

OR

> • ICD-9-CM Principal Diagnosis Code of respiratory failure AND ICD-9-CM Other Diagnosis Codes of pneumonia

Included populations

All pneumonia patients, including patients transferred from a long-term care facility.

Excluded populations

- Patients transferred from another hospital, including another emergency department (ED)
- Patients who had no working diagnosis of pneumonia at the time of admission
- Patients who did not receive antibiotics during hospitalization
- Patients who received *comfort measures only*
- Patients younger than 18 years of age
- Patients whose initial antibiotic was administered more than 36 hours from the time of arrival
- Patients who have received antibiotics within 24 hours prior to hospital arrival

Data was collected with the assistance of the quality department, which performed retrospective reviews. However, the ED also established concurrent measures based on preprinted pneumonia admitting orders. The orders, which reminded the physician of the preferred antibiotics approved by the infection control committee, also included information about time of arrival, time of diagnosis, time of antibiotic order, and time of antibiotic administration. Although only the first and the last data elements were included as part of the official, hospital-wide measure, the intermediate data points (time of diagnosis and order) would be helpful in studying the internal ED processes to improve performance.

The charge nurse was assigned the responsibility of making sure the right antibiotic order sheet was used and that required information was completed. The charge nurse also followed up when clear delays became evident.

Case study #2: Reconciliation of medications

The ED was asked to do its part in meeting the JCAHO's 2005 National Patient Safety Goal regarding reconciliation of medications. The goal requires the hospital to develop a system for reconciling medications at the time of admission and at the time of discharge or transfer. The JCAHO is not clear as to how this goal will be applied to quick turnaround time units like the ED. Therefore, the ED manager felt it important to become involved early in the development process to ensure that the ultimate system account for the realities of the ED.

A subgroup was formed to address medications reconciliation in the ED under the leadership of (and reporting to) the hospital-wide group working on medications reconciliation. The group developed the following system:

✔ A single blue sheet was added to the ED chart with three columns: one for nursing at the time of intake/initial ED assessment; one for the physician during the medical screening examination; and one for both disciplines at the time of discharge, admission, or transfer.

✔ Each column contained a space for known drug allergies and sensitivities, home over-the-counter and prescription medications, and herbal substances routinely taken.

✔ Nursing and medicine obtained the information from the patient and family and recorded it in the appropriate column. Both disciplines were responsible for following up with the other should a discrepancy arise.

✔ The third column was completed at the time of disposition:

• If the patient was discharged home (or to a long-term or assisted-living facility), the physician and discharging nurse ensured that any new discharge medications were reflected in the third column including, when appropriate, instructions about the discontinuation of any previous home medications.

- If the patient were transferred to another general acute-care or psychiatric hospital, any medications given during the stay was reflected in column 3.

- If the patient was admitted to observation or inpatient status, column 3 was left blank and a copy of the form was transmitted to the inpatient pharmacy, along with the admitting orders. The original copy accompanied the patient to the inpatient unit where their process for reconciliation was begun.

This initial design was tested and improved as the hospital developed its overall method of complying with the reconciliation safety goal.

APPENDIX C

Glossary

Glossary

A

Accuracy—The extent to which the measured value of a quantity agrees with the accepted value for that quantity.

Admission percentage—Number of emergency department (ED) admissions divided by the number of ED visits

ADT system—Admission, discharge, and transfer system

Aggregate measure—Combines a standard rule (measure) across several levels of a system.

Attribute—Characteristic of interest.

B

Balancing measures—Additional system standard rules (measures) that might be affected by a measure of interest.

Baseline performance—A set of data that is used for future comparisons.

Benchmarking—A method of comparing ideas, interventions, procedures, and results of a process, system, or operation under study with a similar process, system, or operation that is generally recognized as outstanding. It is intended that the operation under study exceed or at least meet the standards of the model with which it is compared.

Bias—Any difference between the average of a series of measurements and the accepted standard value. Bias is also called systematic error. Increasing sample size will not reduce bias. A measurement system with an acceptable level of bias in called "unbiased."

Boarders hours—Total number of hours admitted inpatients remained in the ED beyond 90 minutes.

C

CMS—Center for Medicare & Medicaid Services.

Calibration—The comparison of a set of measurements to an accepted or standard value for the purpose of detecting or correcting any bias in the measurement process or for establishing a relationship between the measurements and the standard or accepted values.

Collective data—Recorded observations that are aggregated across several levels, such as patients, offices, departments, etc.

Common causes of variation—Elements that are inherent in the process over time, affect everyone working in the process, and affect all outcomes of the process.

Confounding—When the information between two or more variables is combined such that it cannot be separated.

Control chart—A graph with control limits displayed. These limits help the user detect special causes.

Cost of a measure—The resources required to conduct a measurement. This characteristic is important in comparing alternative measurement systems.

D

Data—Recorded observation.

Data capture rate—The number of data points completed divided by the total number of data points.

Data collection and reporting system—The process of gathering information or facts and displaying them so that they are easy to use.

Data collection form—Charts that allow you to simply and systematically collect the recorded observation you want.

Diversion hours—Sum number of hours paramedics were diverted from the ED due to saturation (lack of available beds or staff)

Deselecting measures—Dropping standard rules (measures) that are no longer being used for any sort of decision or action.

E

EMTALA—Emergency Medical Treatment and Active Labor Act.

F

Front-end problems—Process-related issues from patient arrival to bed placement.

G, H, I

Inpatient occupancy—Number of occupied beds divided by the number of available beds

Interval data—Recorded observations using a continuous scale such as a weight measurement of 3.21 grams.

J, K, L

Limit of detection—The lowest concentration level that can be determined to be statistically different from background noise or a "blank" material.

Linearity—The degree to which the calibration of a measurement system can be accomplished with a straight line. A nonlinear system requires more complex calibration procedures.

LCL—Lower control limit.

LOS—Length of stay.

LWBS—Left without being seen, or patients who leave the department prior to discharge.

M

Measurement—A process made up of a combination of procedures, equipment, and personnel. The output of this process is data.

Measurement system—System composed of an aim, attribute (condition or characteristic), item being measured, measure, and method of collecting and analyzing the data.

Model for improvement—A standard made up of two components: current knowledge (with three questions) and the plan-do-study-act (PDSA) cycle.

N

Nominal data—Qualitative recorded observations usually using classifications such as gender or medical diagnosis.

O

Outcome measure—A standard rule (measure) made on the outcome from a person, process, or system.

P

PDSA cycle—The plan-do-study-act cycle is an adaptation of the scientific method and is used as a model for learning and improvement.

Precision—A degree of agreement among independent measurements of a quantity under specified conditions. Precision refers to the ability of a measurement process to reproduce its own outcome. Precision is usually defined in terms of the criteria for repeatability and reproducibility. A measurement process with an acceptable level of precision is called "precise."

Proportion—Measure consisting of a numerator of the number of some characteristic of interest divided by a total population of interest. An example is mortality, which is the number of deaths divided by the number of discharges and transfers. Often proportions are multiplied by 100 to convert to percent.

Q

Qualitative data—Data that cannot be represented with numbers such as pictures, video, or classifications.

Quantitative data—Data that can be represented with numbers.

R

Rate—Measure consisting of a numerator of the number of events over a specified time divided by the population at risk for that event over time.

Reference standard—A material or measurement method that has an accepted value of a unit of measurement. The reference standard can be either a reference material or a reference method.

Regression techniques—A statistical method that establishes an equation (using the method of least squares) between two or more variables.

Reliability—Ability of a measurement system to perform under stated conditions for a stated period of time. In healthcare and in the social sciences, reliability is often used to describe the concept of precision.

Repeatability—Variation in measurements obtained under the best conditions. This often means measurements taken with one instrument, by one person, and in the same time period.

Reproducibility—Variation in measurements obtained by measuring the same item under normal operating conditions. These conditions would reflect the normal work situation: different people, environmental conditions, set-up methods, calibration, etc.

Robustness—The degree to which a measurement system is immune to modest (and inevitable) departures from the procedures and controls in the methods.

Run chart—A graphical display of a measure (original data or a summary statistic) plotted against the time the measure was made.

S

Sampling—Selecting only a proportion (less than 100%) of the items being measured.

Scorecard—A family of measures providing different perspectives for a more holistic understanding.

Sensitivity—Evaluates the ability of a measurement method to detect small changes in the property being measured.

Simplicity of a measure—Ease of use of the measurement system.

Special causes of variation—Causes that are not part of the process all the time or that don't affect everyone but arise due to specific circumstances.

Speed—The time required to complete a measurement (also referred to as turnaround time).

Spider diagram—A graphical display of multiple measures in a single array (Radar chart). This display allows the user to see all measures in one graph.

Stable measure—The tendency of the standard rule (measure) system to remain in statistical control. A stable system is affected only by common causes of variation, while an unstable system is affected by both common and special causes of variation.

Stable process—A method whose outcomes are affected only by common causes; that is, it is in a state of statistical control. A stable process implies only that the variation is predictable within bounds.

Standard measures—A set of rules agreed upon and used by all.

Standardized forms—A set of charts agreed upon and used by all.

Stratifying data—Dividing recorded observations into groups for comparison purposes. An example of a grouping strategy is demographics on patients.

Surrogate measure—A substitute standard rule (measure) that is related to the original.

Systematic error—A mistake in an experiment or trial that may affect the intervention (or treatment group) and the control group result.

T

TAT—Turnaround times.

Temporary bed spaces—Temporary bed locations for patients used during high census periods. Those locations could be a clinical decision unit, overflow unit, holding unit, etc.

Trigger tool—An instrument used for measuring adverse drug events.

U

UCC—Urgent care center.

UCL—Upper control limit.

Unstable process—A method whose outcomes are affected by both common causes and special causes.

V

Validity—The extent to which a measure reflects only the desired attribute of interest.

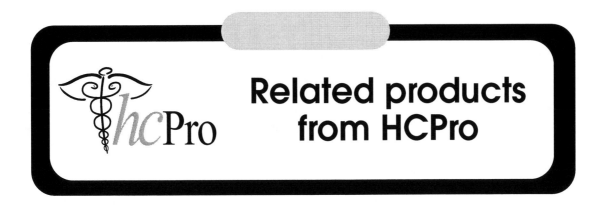

Related products from HCPro

Books

Ready, Set, JCAHO!, Second Edition, ALL NEW Questions, Games, and Other Strategies to Prepare Your Staff for Survey

This new edition reflects the JCAHO's new *Shared Visions—New Pathways*™ survey process and will help you save time and money preparing your staff for survey day. It enables you to put together a schedule of varied training activities for all levels and types of staff that will keep survey preparation fun, interesting, and focused on important key areas. This book includes

- TOOLS, GAMES, EVENTS, and other creative ideas for preparing staff for survey in fun and memorable ways

- Fast-track IDEAS for quick survey prep when you're pressed for time

- JCAHO survey QUESTIONS by focus area that provide hints and examples of compliance and are formatted to be fast and easy handouts for staff training

- Insider tips on how to pass your survey with flying colors from an experienced accreditation expert

The JCAHO Mock Survey Made Simple, 2005 Edition

This just-published version of the popular *The JCAHO Mock Survey Made Simple* book will save you time by assessing your level of compliance with the JCAHO's revamped 2005 requirements and helping you pinpoint which areas of your hospital are in compliance and which areas fall short of the mark.

This way you can effectively channel your hospital's resources and energies into correcting known problem areas instead of wasting time concentrating on issues that don't need additional attention! It is the only resource that actually does the legwork for you, dissecting the JCAHO's *CAMH* and breaking down the information into a series of user-friendly compliance checklists! The detailed checklists cover:

- Accreditation participation requirements

- The National Patient Safety Goals

- Each of the chapters of the *CAMH*

- The most common trouble spots encountered during a JCAHO survey, ranging from restraint and seclusion to the seven environment of care plans

- Self-assessments for the CEO, department managers, medical staff leaders, and front-line staff

Performance Improvement: Winning Strategies for Quality and JCAHO Compliance, Third Edition—Plus CD/ROM

This is the third edition of our award-winning compliance tool! The book and companion CD/ROM have just been updated to reflect the significant changes in the JCAHO's survey process. The JCAHO has revamped its PI standards—specifically around ORYX, FMEA, and core measures—and made PI one of the only remaining planned interviews in the 2004 survey process. You need to know how to respond to the changes to comply! Plus— in addition to keeping PI and quality of care a main focus of its survey process, the JCAHO is adding patient safety as a critical area as well. This book includes a new chapter on patient safety in response to the JCAHO's increased focus on this crucial area, and an educational PowerPoint presentation on CD/ROM.

The JCAHO Survey Coordinator's Handbook, Sixth Edition

The new JCAHO survey process is upon us! Creating a culture of continuous survey readiness is now more important than ever. This how-to compliance tool contains everything you need to know about the new JCAHO requirements and hot-button areas. As with previous editions, this new edition also provides you with field-tested advice, tools—including sample forms and charts—and best practices to help you demonstrate compliance in these critical areas.

Preparing Your Patient Safety Program for JCAHO Survey

Your patient safety program initiatives have never been under more scrutiny than right now. From the JCAHO's new Patient Safety Goals to new survey expectations, you need to make sure your patient safety program is up to par. This book provides you with

- plain-English EXPLANATIONS of the JCAHO's 2004 patient safety standards and step-by-step ADVICE on how to comply with them

- sample CHECKLISTS, FORMS, and DOCUMENTS

- INSIGHT into how your patient safety initiatives will be surveyed

- TIPS and GUIDANCE on implementing a patient safety program, failure modes and effects analysis (FMEA), sentinel events, and root cause analysis

- EXAMPLES of the types of patient safety questions surveyors might ask staff

Quality Measurement: A Practical Guide for the ICU—Plus CD/ROM

Hospitals are always under pressure to measure performance and show quality improvement, and this responsibility often falls to departments. This book will guide the ICU director, nurse manager, or quality improvement director through the process of developing and monitoring appropriate measures for the ICU. It

- discusses specific measures designed for the ICU

- shows how to select measures, collect data, and interpret and present that data

- features case studies, forms, tools, and control charts to overcome common measurement barriers

- provides expert advice from authors Peter Pronovost, MD, PhD, and Ronald Moen, statistical expert

- offers advice on how to analyze your existing measures

The Compliance Guide to the JCAHO's Medication Management Standards

The JCAHO has completely revamped its medication use standards and made medication management one of its new system tracers. During your next survey, JCAHO surveyors will scrutinize your facility's medication policies, procedures, and processes. In this book, an experienced pharmacy director provides you with step-by-step tools and field-tested advice on exactly how to comply with these new requirements. You'll receive plain-English explanations; tools to organize your compliance efforts; specific examples of compliance from real-life hospital pharmacies; and over 35 sample policies, procedures, and forms you can customize for your facility.

CD-ROM

j-mail: JCAHO Survey Prep E-mails for the Whole Staff, 2005 Edition

Under the JCAHO's new survey process, you now need to spend even more time training your staff for survey readiness. This hands-on tool will train ALL staff in a timely and efficient manner. It's an easy-to-use e-mail system designed to help you train your entire staff for survey day. Simple and inexpensive to use, it allows you to reach everyone in your organization with the click of your "Send" button!

This new version of j-mail includes sections of questions on the 2004 survey process, system tracers, patient tracers, general standards, and other tools. In all, you'll receive 48 j-mails—enough for 12 months of weekly e-mails! Each j-mail can be customized to fit your organization's individual needs.

Newsletters

Briefings on JCAHO

This 12-page monthly newsletter is the respected voice of authority for practical, independent guidance on succeeding in the accreditation process at thousands of hospitals nationwide. It will keep you up to speed on all JCAHO changes and provide invaluable insight into how the new JCAHO survey process unfolds. Whether readers are new to surveys or seasoned professionals, each newsletter offers quick reading "how-to" advice on meeting the JCAHO standards. You'll receive tips and information from accreditation experts, including Steve Bryant, that would otherwise cost you dearly in consulting fees and research!

Briefings on Patient Safety

Created exclusively to help health care professionals improve patient safety systems and avoid medical errors, this monthly, 12-page newsletter shares best-practice information regarding medical-error prevention and how to work through damaging circumstances should errors occur. Subscribers get tips on how to perform root-cause analyses, how to inform patients of medical errors, how to involve staff in patient safety initiatives, how to design error-reporting systems, and much, much more.

Briefings on Quality Improvement and Data Reporting

This 12-page monthly resource provides you with the hands-on advice, tools (including data collection forms), and best practices that you need to ensure your hospital scores high on its quality measures and receives all of the Medicare reimbursement it deserves!

Hospital Pharmacy Regulation Report

This 12-page monthly newsletter provides you with the how-to strategies, tips, and tools to comply with today's complex government regulations. We've got your back, whether it's HIPAA, JCAHO, CMS, or ensuring that your pharmacy is adequately staffed. Each month, you and your staff will receive hands-on expert advice, how-to best practices that you can implement immediately, policies and procedures that you can modify to fit your pharmacy, case studies, the latest news and updates from the JCAHO, CMS, and the OIG, and major state pharmacy board news.

To obtain additional information, to order any of the above products, or to comment on *Quality Measurement: A Practical Guide for the Emergency Department*, please contact us at:

Mail:
HCPro
P.O. Box 1168
Marblehead, MA 01945

Toll-free telephone: 800/650-6787
Toll-free fax: 800/639-8511
E-mail: *customerservice@hcpro.com*
Internet: *www.hcmarketplace.com*